英汉对照管理袖珍手册

缓解紧张

Mary Richards　　著
王春艳　　　　　译
Phil Hailstone　　图

U0295920

上海交通大学出版社

图书在版编目(CIP)数据

缓解紧张/(英)理查德兹(Richards,M.)著;王春艳译. —上海:上海交通大学出版社,2002(2011重印)

(英汉对照管理袖珍手册)

ISBN 978-7-313-02866-2

Ⅰ.缓... Ⅱ.①理...②王... Ⅲ.心理卫生-对照读物-英、汉 Ⅳ.R395.6

中国版本图书馆 CIP 数据核字(2001)第 078663 号

责任编辑:汪 俪

英汉对照管理袖珍手册:缓解紧张

王春艳 译

上海交通大学出版社出版发行

(上海市番禺路 951 号 邮政编码 200030)

电话:64071208 出版人:韩建民

立信会计出版社常熟市印刷联营厂 印刷 全国新华书店经销

开本:890mm×1240mm 1/64 印张:3.5 字数:104 千字

2002 年 1 月第 1 版 2011 年 6 月第 5 次印刷

印数:17 201~24 200

ISBN 978-7-313-02866-2/R·033 定价:10.00 元

版权合同登记号：图字：09—2001—428 号

CONTENTS

目 录

INTRODUCTION

INTRODUCTION

WORK & PRESSURE GO HAND IN HAND

There are:

- Deadlines to meet
- Mistakes to rectify
- Demands to satisfy
- Targets to achieve
- Problems to resolve
- Challenges to rise to

You may find:

- Goal posts are moved
- Work is interrupted
- Working relationships become strained
- There is too much or too little to do
- The work stretches you or bores you
- The future of your job is uncertain

Everyone in every job experiences pressure.

工作和压力同时并存

工作中存在着各种压力：
- 有很多任务要在规定期限内完成
- 有很多错误要修改
- 有很多要求要去满足
- 有很多目标要去实现
- 有很多存在的问题要去解决
- 有很多新的挑战要去迎接

你会发现：
- 工作目标总在变化
- 工作不时被打断
- 工作关系变得紧张
- 工作繁多或无事可做
- 工作太累或很枯燥
- 工作前途不稳定

任何人在任何工作中都会遇到压力。

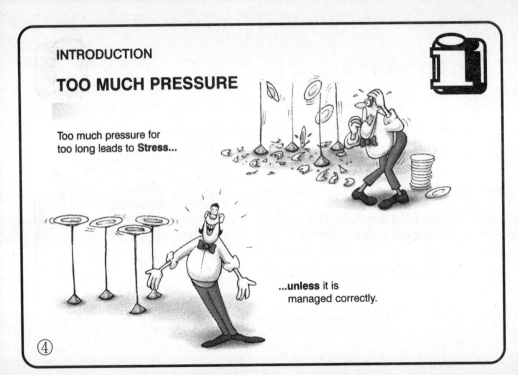

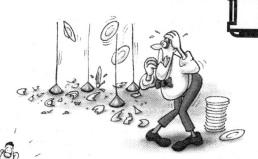

导言
过多的压力

长时间的过多压力会
引起**紧张** ······

······ 除非你能正确地
处理压力

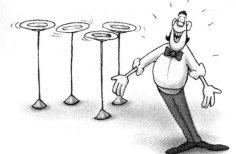

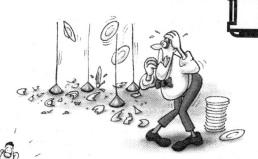

⑤

PRESSURE LEVELS

At one level, pressure may be a positive aid to performance:

- The deadline that spurs you on
- The target that motivates you
- The challenge that inspires you

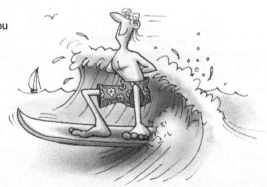

压力的程度

适当的压力对你的工作表现有积极的帮助作用：
- 刺激你按时完成任务
- 驱使你达到既定目标
- 鼓舞你迎接新的挑战

PRESSURE LEVELS

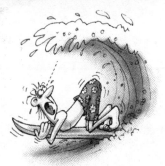

At another level, pressure may trigger a mechanism to tell you that something is wrong and you start to experience stress.

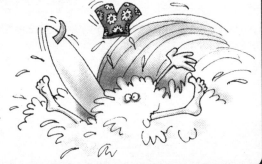

Continue beyond this level for too long and you can seriously damage your mental and physical well-being.

压力的程度

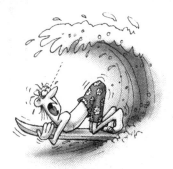

压力达到一定程度,
你就会感觉到不适,
并开始紧张。

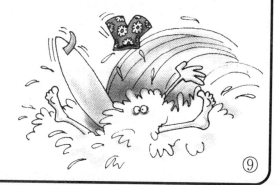

这种状况若长期持续
下去,你的身心健康
会受到严重侵害。

⑨

INTRODUCTION

REALITY OF THE WORLD WE WORK IN

As technology...

- Reshapes jobs
- Increases the speed at which we work
- Makes information and knowledge quickly out of date

...we will all experience more pressure at work.

As markets...

- Demand a more flexible workforce
- Influence the shape of organisations
- Remove the 'job for life'

...we will all experience more pressure at work.

我们所在的现实社会

科技……
- 改变工作的形式
- 加快着工作的节奏
- 使信息和知识很快过时

……因此工作中我们将担负更多的压力。

市场……
- 要求更灵活的劳动生力军
- 影响着组织的形态
- 改变了"一生只做一份工作"的观念

……因此工作中我们将担负更多的压力。

YOU CAN CHOOSE

As the pressure at work increases
you have a choice:

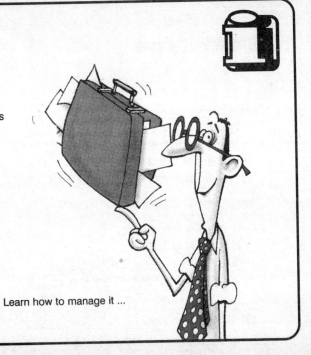

Learn how to manage it ...

⑫

你可以选择

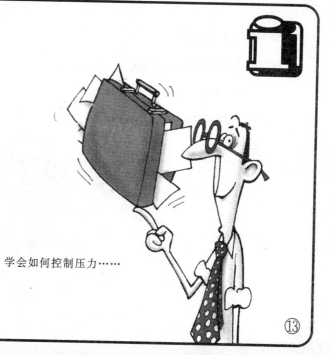

随着工作压力加重，
你可以选择：

学会如何控制压力……

⑬

INTRODUCTION

YOU CAN CHOOSE

... or let work pressures manage you!

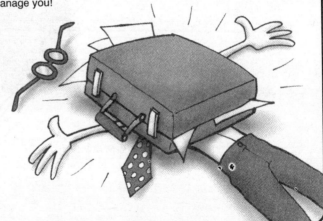

导言
你可以选择

……你也可以选择被压力击垮！

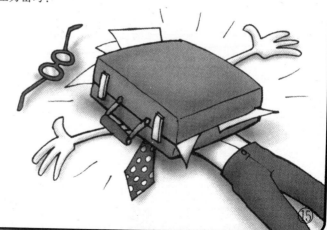

NOTES
笔 记

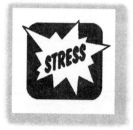

STRESS
紧 张

A DEFINITION OF STRESS

Because stress means different things to different people...

- Tackling a task for the first time
- A meeting with the boss
- Giving a presentation
- A delayed delivery of important supplies
- An irate customer
- A tight deadline
- An unnecessary mistake
- A difference of opinion

...because what's stressful to you today, may not necessarily be stressful to you tomorrow or the day after...

什么是紧张

因为不同的人有不同的紧张……

- 初次尝试完成某项任务
- 要和领导会面
- 当众做口头报告
- 耽误了某项重要的供货任务
- 遇到难对付的客户
- 完成任务的期限很短
- 犯了不该犯的错误
- 持有不同意见

……因为今天使你紧张的东西,明天或将来不一定会令你紧张……

STRESS

A DEFINITION OF STRESS

...because stress can be...

POSITIVE	or	NEGATIVE

- An opportunity to prove yourself

- You work better to a deadline

- It gives you a positive emotional charge or 'high'

- You become less efficient - performance and productivity fall

- Deadlines send you into a blind panic - you achieve nothing

- You seek comfort by snacking, smoking or drinking

...stress is best described as: **an individual's response to pressure.**

紧张
紧张是什么

……因为紧张的作用可以是……

积极的	或	消极的

- 是一次提高自己的机会

- 为了按期完成任务,你会更努力地工作

- 它会使你以更积极、高度的感情投入工作

- 使你变得工作效率低下——业绩和生产率降低

- 过度紧张使你无法按期完成任务———一事无成

- 为了安慰自己,沉溺于吃零食、吸烟或喝酒

……所以对紧张的最佳表述为:**个体对压力的不同反应。**

WHAT HAPPENS INSIDE YOUR BODY?

If you perceive a pressure as a threat or a challenge, your body will automatically go into overdrive:

- Your heart rate increases and your blood pressure rises
- Your muscles harden and tense in readiness for action
- Your digestive process slows and more acid is produced in the stomach
- Your breathing becomes quicker as your lungs try to take up more oxygen

This automatic reaction is often known as the 'fight' or 'flight' response because these changes prepare the body to be able to fight or run away.

你的体内发生了什么

　　如果你把压力看成是威胁和挑战,那么你的身体会自动进入异常状态:
- 心跳加快,血压升高
- 肌肉变得坚硬、紧张,为行动做准备
- 消化变缓,胃里产生过多胃酸
- 呼吸加速,以便吸入更多氧气

　　身体这种自动的反应被称为"迎击或逃离"的反应,因为这些变化都是为了使身体进入迎击或逃离的准备状态。

USEFUL CYCLE OR DOWNWARD SPIRAL?

The fight or flight response was a very appropriate mechanism for primitive man. Being able to fight or run to safety when under pressure ensured his survival.
It was a useful cycle.

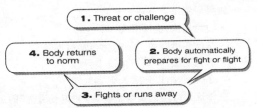

1. Threat or challenge

2. Body automatically prepares for fight or flight

3. Fights or runs away

4. Body returns to norm

However, try applying this cycle to your work environment.

You feel threatened or challenged by pressures at work. The fight or flight response is triggered. Your body goes into overdrive. Neither fighting nor running away does much for your career prospects. So you don't. You are now under more pressure both mentally and physically. You continue to ignore the fight or flight cycle and, as a consequence, the pressures increase. You have unwittingly converted a useful cycle into a downward spiral.

紧张

有用的循环还是恶性发展？

　　迎击或逃离的反应是原始人具
有的正常机能。遇到压力能够正面
迎击或反身逃开，才能保障自己的
生存。这个过程是一个有用的循环。

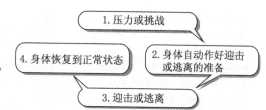

1. 压力或挑战

2. 身体自动作好迎击
或逃离的准备

4. 身体恢复到正常状态

3. 迎击或逃离

　　但是，在工作环境中应用这个过程时，会遇到另一种情况。工作中遇到压力，感受到
威胁和挑战，于是便触发了迎战或逃离反应，身体进入一种过度紧张状态。但对你的前
途来讲，迎战或逃离都不会有很多的帮助，于是你什么也不去做，这时精神和身体上就有
了更大的压力。你若仍然不运用迎击或逃离反应的循环，压力会继续加重。你不明智地
把一个有用的循环变成了恶性发展。

㉕

THE TRIGGER

The key to understanding and managing stress is to know that the fight or flight response is only activated when you perceive a pressure as a threat or challenge. Think about it:

Your boss asks you to meet in Room 4 in half an hour. **If** your response is to start to think...

- What have I done wrong?
- Am I going to be fired?
- Why Room 4?
- Why me?

...you will trigger the fight or flight response. You become so concerned about the meeting that you can think of little else. Consequently, you waste half an hour and in doing so increase the pressure on yourself. You will arrive at the meeting in a state of stress.

紧张

紧张的导火索

　　理解和控制压力的关键是要意识到当压力被视为威胁和挑战的时候,会引起迎击或逃离反应。

　　设想你的老板要你半个小时后到四号房间见他,如果你马上想到:

- 我做错了什么?
- 我会被解雇吗?
- 为什么要在四号房间见我?
- 为什么要见我?

　　……这样你就会产生迎击或逃离的反应。因为你太在意这个会面,其他事情就考虑不进去了。结果是你浪费了半个小时想这些问题并增加了自己的压力。当你去和老板会面的时候,心中肯定充满了紧张。

SOURCE OF STRESS

There are many pressures at work, but there is only one source of stress. **You.**

Check it out for yourself. Think of a stressful situation at work. Ask yourself the following questions:

- What is creating the pressure in this situation?
- What is the response to the pressure in this situation?
- Who is responding?
- Where, therefore, is the source of stress?

Because stress is an individual's response to pressure, you will always be the source of your own stress. Your stress will be the result of your own response to the pressures you experience at work.

紧张的原因

　　工作中有各种压力,但引起紧张的原因只有一个,那就是**你自己**。

　　看看自己是不是属于这种情况。设想一下工作中的紧张状态,问问自己下列问题:

- 什么引起了工作压力?
- 对这种压力的反应是什么?
- 谁在做出反应?
- 那么,紧张来自何处?

　　因为紧张是个体对压力的不同反应,引起紧张的原因只有你自己。紧张是你自己对工作中压力的个人反应。

WHERE MIGHT PRESSURES AT WORK COME FROM?

The physical environment: noise; overcrowding; uncomfortable working conditions; lack of parking facilities.

The characteristics of the job: repetitive work; tight deadlines; shift work; too much or too little to do; too much or too little responsibility; travel; long or anti-social hours; responding to emergencies.

The organisation's culture: being in a minority (male/female; smoking/non-smoking; etc); rules, regulations and expectations; level of stability or tendency to change.

The people (management, staff, suppliers, customers, shareholders, you): relationships with others at work; not being the right person for the job; being too demanding of yourself and others; being a 'yes' person; inefficient work habits.

紧张

工作中的压力来自何方？

　　外部环境：噪音，拥挤，恶劣的工作条件，停车设施缺乏等等。

　　工作特性：重复的工作，完成任务的期限很短，工作不断变换，工作繁重或无事可做，责任过重或过轻，工作需要外出，社交时间过多或由于工作无法社交，负责处理突发紧急事件等等。

　　组织文化：处于一个少数群体（男性/女性，吸烟/不吸烟等等）之中，规章、条例和期望，稳定的程度和变化的趋势。

　　人的因素（管理人员、全体员工、供应商、客户、股东和你自己）：工作中与其他人之间的关系，工作不适合自己，对自己和别人过分苛求，在任何情况下都说"是"，没有效率的工作习惯。

STRESS

HOW TO RECOGNISE STRESS

Your response to a pressure may result in stress, but how will you recognise it? Although physiologically we all react in a similar way (rise in heart rate, tense muscles, etc) our overt reactions and behaviours may be very different. These are just a few of the many signs you might see, hear or feel:

- **SEE:** nail biting; twitching eye/eyebrow; frequent licking or biting of lips; excessive blinking; a change in eating or drinking patterns from abstinence to over-indulgence; signs of tiredness; crying...

- **HEAR:** slamming of doors, phones, papers or fists on desks; unusually rapid speech; drumming of fingers; emotional outbursts; swearing; unco-ordinated speech; jingling of coins or keys; pen top flicking; sighing...

- **FEEL:** sweaty; clammy; flushed; tense; frustrated; angry; isolated; hopeless; impatient; irritable; depressed; anxious; stretched; challenged...

紧张
如何意识到紧张

    对压力的反应会导致紧张,但如何知道自己处于紧张状态了呢?尽管生理上的反应(如心跳加快、肌肉紧张等等)都是相同的,但每个人的外在的明显的反应和行为是不同的。下面是一些你能看到、听到或感觉到的紧张的表现:

    • **看到的**:咬指甲,眼睛或眉毛抽动,频繁地舔咬嘴唇,总是眨眼,打破原来的节制,过度进食、饮酒,劳累的迹象,哭泣⋯⋯

    • **听到的**:猛地关门,把电话、纸张或拳头敲在桌子上的声音,不寻常的语速加快,手指不停地敲桌子,情感突然迸发,咒骂,说话不连贯,丁当地摆弄硬币或钥匙,轻敲笔尖,叹气⋯⋯

    • **感到的**:流汗,冷淡,脸红,紧张,失意,愤怒,孤独,失望,急躁,易怒,压抑,焦虑,懒散,感到挑战⋯⋯

HEED SIGNS OF STRESS

Stress is a downward spiral that can seriously damage your mental and physical well-being.

Fortunately, your body will give you signs that you are stressed. These signs are the results of your thoughts and responses to pressure. **Heed them.**

留心紧张的表现

　　紧张呈一种恶性发展的趋势,它对你的精神和身体健康都会造成伤害。

　　幸运的是当你紧张时,身体会有所表现。这些表现就是你的想法和对压力的反应。

对这些一定要警觉。

NOTES

笔 记

㊱

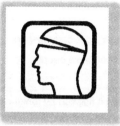

YOUR THOUGHTS

你 的 想 法

THE FACTS

When your thoughts trigger stress, your body responds:

'I can't possibly stand up in front of those people'
You break out in a cold sweat

'The boss will kill me if I don't get it finished by tonight'
Your stomach begins to churn

Controlling your thoughts will help you to
control your responses. This will reduce
your stress.

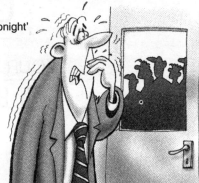

你的想法
一些事实

当你的思想纵容紧张时,身体会产生相应的反应:
当你想到"在那么多人面前我肯定站不起来"时,肯定会突然浑身冒冷汗。
"我要是今晚做不完,老板会杀了我。"一想到此,你的胃就开始痉挛。
控制你的思想会帮你控制对紧张的反应,这样会减轻紧张的程度。

THE PROOF & CONSEQUENCES

Prove to yourself that your body responds to your thoughts. Watch a film or read a book. If the story is frightening, you will feel your pulse racing. If the story is sad, the tears will start to flow.

Now consider the consequences of this at work. If, for example, you really think that you're going to lose your job, your body will start to behave as though you've already lost it.

How do your thoughts affect your behaviour at work? Are they generating pressure and stress, or are they reducing it?

你的想法

验证和后果

　　自己验证一下思想对身体的反应有影响这个事实。当你看电影或看书时,如果故事情节很吓人,你会感到心跳加快;如果故事令人悲伤,你往往会流泪。

　　现在想一想这一事实在工作中会造成的后果。假如你真的认为自己会丢掉现在的工作,那么你的身体会表现得好像你已经失去了这份工作的样子。

　　你的思想是如何影响你在工作中的表现的? 它们是产生压力还是减轻压力呢?

PERSPECTIVES INFLUENCE RESULT

Some perspectives generate stress. Others don't.

Imagine that a new software program is going to be installed on your computer at work. You might think:

- New software probably means job losses; you're worried
- It'll take me twice as long to get the work done; you're frustrated
- Thank goodness the company's joining the 21st century; you're relieved
- Great, it's an opportunity to add another skill to my CV; you're enthusiastic

How you respond to a pressure depends on your perspective.

你的想法
不同的想法产生不同的结果

有些想法会引起紧张,有些则不会。

假设你所在的公司决定在你的电脑上装一套新软件,你也许会有以下想法:

• 新的软件有可能意味着失业;你很担心

• 和以前相比,完成同样的工作需要两倍的时间;你感到灰心

• 感谢上帝,公司进入了 21 世纪;你如释重负

• 太棒了,这是一个好机会,使你能在自己的简历上增加一项技能;你热情高涨

对压力做出什么样的反应是由你的观点决定的。

YOUR THOUGHTS

INFLUENCE & CHOICE

Your perspective may be influenced by:

- Previous experience of a situation; did you survive, how did you manage then?
- Being faced with something for the first time; fear of the unknown, no previous experience to draw on.
- What else is going on in your life; nothing much or the straw that breaks the camel's back.
- How you feel at that particular time; on top of the world or positively steam rollered.
- Whether you are alone or supported by others; being isolated or being able to share your concerns.
- Your beliefs and values; that people should be treated equally, that your home life is more important than your work.
- Your personality; type A (competitive, high achieving, restless) or type B (more easy going, more relaxed).

Your perspective may be influenced, but you are still free to make choices. Who tells you whether to laugh at a joke or not? You may be influenced, but the choice is yours.

你的想法
影响和选择

你对问题的观点可能会受下列因素的影响：

• 以前经历过的事情；当时你是否克服了困难？困难是如何被克服的？

• 初次遇到某件事；对未知事物的恐惧，没有关于此事的经验。

• 生活其他方面的进展情况；没什么大不了的还是有致命因素存在？

• 某个特定时间的感觉；是兴高采烈还是垂头丧气？

• 自己单打独斗还是有人帮忙；孤立于他人还是能向别人倾诉你的烦恼？

• 你的信仰和价值观；如人人平等，家庭比工作更重要。

• 你的个性；是 A 类性格（有竞争力，成就高，不安分）还是 B 类性格（容易相处，较放松）？

你的观点会受到以上诸多因素的影响，但你的最终决定还是由你自己做出。听到幽默后没人会告诉你该不该笑，你可能会受到其他因素的影响，但最终做出决定的还是你自己。

CHOOSING YOUR PERSPECTIVE

Learning to adjust and choose pressure-reducing thoughts and perspectives may take a little practice.

- Generate different perspectives by:
  - **Writing** the facts of the situation down on paper; it will clarify your thinking and help you to see the situation in different ways.
  - **Putting** yourself in the shoes of others. How might they perceive the situation?
  - **Talking** to others. Other people will always be able to help you find a different perspective. You don't have to agree with them, but they may open your mind to even more ideas.
- Assess each perspective in terms of whether it will generate more or less pressure.
- Choose the one that will reduce your pressure.

你的想法
选择你的观点

学会调节、选择合适的减轻压力的想法和观点,需要做一些练习。

• 通过以下途径,可以产生不同观点:

- **写**　把遇到的情景写下来;它会帮你理清思路,从不同的角度看问题。

- **假设**　假设你是别人,他们会怎么处理这种情况呢?

- **讲**　把你的问题讲给别人听。别人往往会帮你发现不同的观点,你不必一定要同意他们的说法,但他们会使你开拓思路,找到更多观点。

• 对每个观点进行评判,看它是加剧还是减轻压力。

• 选定能减轻你压力的观点。

YOUR THOUGHTS

PUTTING IT IN PERSPECTIVE

When you can only think of perspectives that increase the pressure:

- **Imagine the worst.** Think how the situation might be worse than it really is. It will enable you to view your original thoughts in a better light and it will put you under less pressure. Try it. Things will not be as bad as they seemed at first.

- **Check your values.** Are you becoming stressed about something that in the bigger picture of life is not really that significant at all? What's really important to you in life? Don't stress yourself with less important things.

你的想法
换个角度看问题

当你甩不掉使压力增加的观点时:

• **假设最坏的结果**。设想情况最坏会坏到什么样。这样会让你用一种稍轻松的观点去审视你原来的思想,从而缓解自己的压力。试一试,你会看到事情并不像起初想象的那样糟。

• **核实自己的价值观**。想一想自己是不是在为一些从长远角度来看并不重要的小事而紧张压抑?而人生中真正重要的事情是什么?别让不重要的事束缚我们,为它而紧张。

BEYOND YOUR CONTROL?

Rumours of redundancy, company take-overs and changes in business legislation are all situations where you may be under pressure because you **feel** that you have no control. You blame the management, the system or fate. Your thoughts confirm your helplessness. They generate stress.

Don't concern yourself with things that are out of your control. Focus instead on what is within your control. If, for example, you think you might be made redundant, make sure that given the choice the company would want to keep you; get your CV up to date, study and practise interview techniques.

In every situation there is always something within your control. Start with controlling your thoughts. They will deliver controlled responses.

你的想法
超出了控制范围?

　　听到裁员的谣言,公司被接管,以及商业法规的变化等等都会使你紧张,因为你**感到**无法控制这些事件。于是你就抱怨管理状况、整个机制或命运。你的想法证实了你的无助。它们产生了压力。

　　不要去理睬那些你无法控制的东西,把主要精力放在你能控制的事情上。假如你认为自己有可能被裁掉,那么你应该争取让公司认为你有用而留住你;使你的简历保持常新,学习并练习面试技巧。

　　在任何情况下,总会有一些事情在你的控制范围之内。首先要做的是控制你的思想,这样才能在反应时有所控制。

CONTROLLING YOUR THOUGHTS

When you are under pressure you may find that:

- You can't think straight
- You can't focus on the job in hand
- Your thoughts run away with you

Try controlling your thoughts by focusing your mind. Hang a favourite picture on your wall; keep on your desk a photo that makes you happy; write a poem or short piece of text you enjoy in your diary. Focus on them when your thoughts are out of control. Use them as anchors to bring your thoughts into line, and put you back in control.

Practise it. If you use the same anchor all the time it will set a pattern in your mind. As the pattern establishes, you will be able to take control of your thoughts more quickly.

你的思想
控制你的思想

有压力时你会发现:
- 不能冷静而有条理地思考
- 不能集中精力干手头的工作
- 总是走神

通过集中精力来控制自己的思想。在墙上挂上自己喜欢的图片,在书桌上摆上能让自己开心的照片,在日记里写下你喜欢的诗或散文。当思路烦乱无法控制时,你就可以把精力集中在这些喜欢的东西上,把它们看成是你思想归航的锚,进而把你从烦恼中拉出来,让思想步入正轨。

不妨练习一下这个方法。如果经常练习,脑子里就会形成一种定势。这种定势一旦形成,你就能更快地控制你的思想。

YOUR THOUGHTS

THOUGHTS INTO WORDS

Your thoughts are reinforced by what you say, so try:

- **Self-talk:** repeat your thoughts over and over in your head; it will reinforce your belief and your commitment

- **Saying it out loud:** share your thoughts with others - it will strengthen your resolve; going public with your thoughts is a great way to make you stick to them

Putting your thoughts into words helps to make your thoughts a reality. Remember, thoughts influence responses.

把思想变成语言

　　语言可以强化思想,所以你不妨试一试下列方法:
　　• **自言自语**:在脑子里一遍一遍地重复自己的想法,它会加强你的信仰和行为。
　　• **大声讲述**:把你的想法讲给别人听,这样会加强决心,把你的想法公开是使你坚持这样做下去的一个非常好的方法。
　　把你的思想变为语言可以帮你把思想变成现实。切记:思想影响反应。

NOTES
笔 记

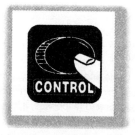

YOUR RESPONSES

你 的 反 应

YOUR RESPONSE, YOUR STRESS, YOUR CHOICE

Realising that stress comes from your thoughts and responses can be quite sobering. However, it can also be liberating:

- You can choose your thoughts and responses; you may be influenced, but ultimately the choice is yours
- You can control your thoughts and responses; it may take effort, time and even practice, but they are yours to control

Exercise this choice. Take control. Reduce your stress.

你的反应
你的反应,你的紧张,你的选择

　　意识到紧张来自你的思想和反应会让你觉得沉重,但是,它也会给你选择和控制的自由:

　　•你可以选择自己的思想和反应;虽然你可能会受到别人的影响,但最终的选择还是由你做出。

　　•你可以控制自己的思想和反应;做到这一点需要努力、时间和练习,但它们是在你的控制范围之内的。

　　练习如何选择。施加控制。减轻压力。

RESPONDING TO PRESSURE

Responses to pressure vary from person to person and from pressure to pressure.
They may depend on what else is actually happening at the time or how you're feeling.

Amongst others, your response may be:

Physical - 'butterflies' in your stomach, headaches, shallow breathing...

Mental - forgetfulness, lack of concentration, worry...

Emotional - quarrelsome, defensive, embarrassed...

Behavioural - too busy for anything other than work, drink/smoke more than usual, insomnia...

How do **you** respond to the pressures at work? Use some of the ideas on the following pages to help control your responses to the pressures of time, workload, change, people, conflict and you.

对压力的反应

　　不同的人对同一种压力有不同的反应,同一个人对不同的压力也会有不同的反应。对压力的反应还要看当时的状况和你的感受。

　　你的反应可能会表现在以下几个方面:

　　身体上——紧张得恶心;头疼;呼吸短促……

　　精神上——健忘,注意力不集中,担心……

　　感情上——易吵,易怒,困窘……

　　行为上——除了工作,没有心思顾及其他,过度吸烟、饮酒,失眠……

　　面对工作中的压力,**你**又如何做出反应呢? 以下几页提供了一些方法,你可以利用它们来帮助自己控制面对来自时间、工作重负、变化、人、矛盾和你自身的各方面的反应。

PRESSURE OF TIME

Time is one of the greatest pressures at work.
How do you respond to it?

- Not enough time   - panic
- Wasted time   - annoyance; guilt
- Interrupted time   - frustration; impatience
- Not giving enough time   - concern; worry
- Not being on time   - anxiety
- Too much time   - boredom

These responses are all signs of stress.
You may experience them many times
in each day.

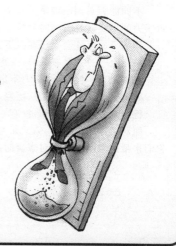

你的反应
时间的压力

时间是工作上遇到的最大的压力之一。

你该如何做出反应呢？

- 时间不够用　　　　　　　　——惊慌
- 浪费了时间　　　　　　　　——烦恼,负罪感
- 被打断的工作时间　　　　　——受挫,不耐烦
- 没有给出足够时间　　　　　——挂念,担心
- 未能准时　　　　　　　　　——焦虑
- 时间过多　　　　　　　　　——枯燥

这些反应都是紧张的表现,你可能每天都会遇到很多次这样的情况。

PRESSURE OF TIME

MAKING IT WORSE

You will always be under a certain amount of pressure from time because it's a limited resource. But do you make the pressure worse than it need be? Do you:

- Always stop what you're doing to help others?
- Open the post as soon as it arrives?
- Work to unrealistic deadlines?
- Spend a disproportionate amount of time dotting the i's and crossing the t's?
- Watch the clock?
- Write and rewrite lengthy 'To Do' lists?
- Under-estimate the time you need?
- Work through the day without any breaks?
- Busy yourself with the tasks that interest or flatter you?
- Arrive late for meetings?
- Spend most of your day dealing with phone calls and other interruptions?
- Allow one delay at the beginning of your day to snowball into your whole schedule so that you end up chasing your tail?

Doing any of these things will increase the pressure you're under.

你的反应
时间的压力
使压力加重

　　因为时间是有限的资源,所以工作中总会遇到时间上的某种压力。检查一下你的下列做法,是否使压力加重了?
- 经常停下自己手头的事情去帮助别人?
- 邮件一到,马上打开?
- 为满足不现实的工作期限而拼命工作?
- 对细节问题花费过多的时间?
- 总是看表?
- 总是不停地写出并修改冗长的"任务"清单?
- 低估完成任务所需的时间?
- 整天埋头工作不休息?
- 忙于自己感兴趣或能满足自己虚荣心的工作?
- 开会迟到?
- 一天的工作时间很多时候用于接电话或其他干扰上?
- 一开始便延误工作,接下去使任务每一步都往后拖,最后只好赶进度,瞎忙?

上述任何一种状况都会增加你的压力。

PRESSURE OF TIME

WAYS TO REDUCE THE PRESSURE

Try reducing the pressure you're under by:

- Applying the Pareto principle to your list of tasks (20% of the tasks will give you 80% of your results); identify those key tasks and make them a priority

- Distinguishing between urgent tasks (crisis, unplanned, demands, etc) and important tasks (that achieve your prime objectives, give you maximum return for effort)

- Being selective; not all tasks need 'polishing'

- Planning uninterrupted time; divert your phone; make it known that you are unavailable

时间的压力
减轻压力的方法

通过以下方法,可以减轻你的压力:

• 在列任务清单时,运用帕累托原则(完成 20％的任务会给你带来 80％的收获),找出最重要的任务,着手先去解决它们

• 区分紧急任务(危机、意外需求等等)和重要任务(帮你达到首要目的、对你的付出能给以最大回报的任务)

• 有选择性地工作;并不是所有的工作都需要精雕细琢

• 留出不被打断的工作时间;把你的电话转开,让别人知道你很忙,没时间接电话

YOUR RESPONSES

PRESSURE OF TIME

WAYS TO REDUCE THE PRESSURE (Cont'd)

- Saying 'no' to 'urgent' requests, interruptions and unreasonable demands
- Planning to do the most demanding tasks when you're at your best
- Setting realistic deadlines for tasks and sticking to them; when necessary, re-negotiate deadlines as soon as possible
- Working together; if you have the authority, delegate; alternatively, think about asking others for help; who would do your job if you were away?

时间的压力

减轻压力的方法(续)

- 敢于对"紧急"请求、总打断你工作的事和无礼的要求说"不"
- 做好计划,把最困难的工作放在你精力最充沛的时间去做
- 给任务设定切实可行的期限,并严格依照其执行。必要时,对任务的期限及时进行修改
- 与他人合作;如果你有分配任务的权力,把任务分配出去;否则可以考虑一下请求他人的帮助;你不在岗的时候,谁会来替你做工作呢?

PRESSURE OF WORK

When you've got too much or too little to do at work do you:

- Blame others?
- Complain, gripe or groan?
- Work every hour available or do nothing?
- Worry that you'll lose your job?

Negative thoughts and responses will only add to your pressure. They will take you down the spiral of stress. Try to stop them. Replace them with more constructive thoughts and responses.

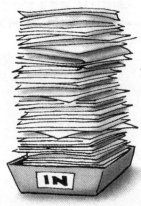

你的反应
工作的压力

当你工作任务过重或过轻时,你是否会:
- 责怪他人?
- 抱怨、愤怒还是呻吟?
- 不停地工作,还是什么也不做?
- 担心丢掉工作?

消极的思想和反应会加重你的压力,不断增加的压力会把你卷入紧张的漩涡。要设法阻止这种趋势,用积极的想法和反应取代消极的想法和反应。

PRESSURE OF WORK

CONSTRUCTIVE RESPONSES

When you've got too much work, stop. Establish the real reason for your excessive workload. Maybe you need to:

- Plan ahead for known increases in workload (end of month duties; seasonal peaks; people on leave; etc)
- Be less of a perfectionist
- Start delegating or delegate more effectively
- Work more efficiently
- Balance your tasks - mix those you like with those you don't like; the long with the short; the difficult with the easy
- Focus on one task at a time
- Be more proactive rather than reactive
- Talk to someone to get a different perspective and new ideas about how to manage your workload
- Stop worrying and start doing
- Put the tips on pages 66~69 into practice

你的反应
工作的压力
积极的反应

当面临过多的工作任务时,应该停下来。找出你工作负担过重的原因。也许你需要:

• 事先做计划,防备可预期的工作上的繁忙情况(比如每月月底,季节性高峰期,有人离岗等等)
• 不要对每件事都追求尽善尽美
• 尝试把任务委派给别人并使委派变得更有效
• 更有效率地工作
• 平衡自己的工作,把喜欢的和不喜欢的工作搭配着做,需要时间长的和需要时间短的工作、难完成的和容易完成的搭配着做
• 每次集中精力做一项工作
• 积极主动的态度总比消极应对的态度要好
• 向别人讲出你的任务,可以得到如何来对付重任的不同的观点和想法
• 停止担心,开始行动
• 把第 66～69 页提到的建议付诸实施

WHEN THERE'S NOT ENOUGH TO DO

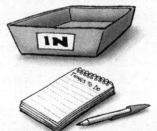

Try to:

- Look for ways to contribute. Who is rushed off their feet? How could you help them? Offer to do tasks that are well within your grasp - phone screening, photocopying, fetching and delivering. Helping out just once normally leads to work coming your way a second time.

- Set yourself deadlines, goals and challenges to give yourself enough pressure to get moving. Perhaps you can do a task with greater accuracy than before.

- Generate ideas on how to increase your workload by talking to others.

- Check your job specification. Are you doing everything you're supposed to do? Discuss it with your boss.

你的反应
当工作量少时

　　你不妨尝试以下做法：
　　• 找出可以做贡献的方法。看看谁正忙得不可开交？你怎样才能帮助他们？主动去帮别人做些你力所能及的事情，比如说，筛选电话，复印，拿取或转送物件等等。一旦你主动帮着做了这些事，下次有此类工作时，他们会主动找你来做。
　　• 给自己定一个完成任务的最后期限、目标和挑战。这样可以给自己一些压力，进而使自己行动起来。也许你会获得比以前更高的准确率。
　　• 把你的状况讲给别人听，看是否可以得到其他建议，增加你的工作量。
　　• 核实自己的工作规范。你是否把每项该做的事都做了？和老板讨论一下你的情况。

RESPONDING TO CHANGE

When faced with change you will go through the following process:

- **Awareness** How will this affect me?
- **Shock** They're going to do what? I can't believe it.
- **Denial** There's no way this'll work. It'll blow over.
- **Frustration** If it wasn't for the management...
- **Realisation** If that's what's going to happen then...
- **Acceptance** If you can't beat them, join them.
- **Adaptation** It could be worse. At least it means that...
- **Integration** The change becomes the norm. There's nothing to react to.

Regardless of the change, be it positive or negative, you will go through all of these stages. However, the speed at which you go through them will vary from change to change and from person to person.

你对变化的反应

    面临变化时,你会经历下述过程:
- **知道**:变化将怎样影响到我?
- **震惊**:他们打算做什么? 我简直不敢相信。
- **否定**:这样根本行不通。会把整个计划搞砸。
- **沮丧**:要不是为了管理的需要……
- **意识到**:如果它真的会发生,那么……
- **接受**:如果不能阻止它,那么投入变化。
- **适应**:情况本来可能会更糟,至少它意味着……
- **融合**:变化成了常规,没有什么可反对的。

    不管变化是积极的还是消极的,你都会经历这些过程。但是你经历这几步的速度会因变化不同而不同,也会因人而异。

RESPONDING TO CHANGE

REDUCING THE PRESSURE

All stages of the change process are likely to put you under pressure, but some more than others. To reduce the pressure try:

- Asking questions - seek as much information as possible; you may be rejecting the change before you understand the full story

- Being as open-minded as possible - for every negative you identify, find a positive

- Moving with the change as quickly as possible - while it is important to question change and not 'blindly' accept it, the quicker you move with rather than against it, the sooner pressure will be reduced

- Sharing your concerns with others - being alone with change will increase the pressure you're under; talking with others will help you see things from different perspectives

你的反应
对变化的反应
减轻压力

　　在经历变化的这几个阶段中,你都会感到有压力存在,但压力的程度轻重不一。要想减轻压力,不妨试下列方法:

　　• 问问题——寻求尽可能多的信息。没有了解到事情的全部真相时,你有可能对变化持有抵触情绪

　　• 尽可能做一个开放的人——对任何一个你发现的缺点,争取找一个优点

　　• 尽可能快地随着变化而调整自己——虽然对变化提出质疑,不盲目接受是好事,但是你能越快随着变化而改变自己,而不是一味的抵触,你就能越快摆脱自己的压力

　　• 把自己的担心讲给别人听——自己一个人承受变化会增加你的压力;和别人谈一谈会帮你从不同角度来看问题

INTRODUCING CHANGE

When you introduce change to others, reduce the pressure they're under by:

- Giving them time to come to terms with the thought of change; avoid surprises
- Where possible, introducing the change as an idea, a topic for discussion rather than a fait accompli
- Involving them as much as possible at all stages of the change; if they are involved, they will own it and be more positive about the change
- Talking to them about how they feel; when people have a voice it gives them a sense of control, reducing the pressure they're under
- Giving them as much information as possible; stress is often caused by people drawing their own conclusions through lack of information

你的反应
让别人接受变化

    当你让别人接受变化的时候,可以通过以下方法帮助别人减轻压力:
    • 要想让别人接受变化,需要给出足够时间让他逐步接受,不要给人突然袭击
    • 可能的话,使变化成为一个讨论的主题或观点而不是既定的事实
    • 创造条件,让他们参与变化的每一个阶段;如果参与了每个阶段,他们会视自己为创造变化的人,进而对它持积极态度
    • 和他们谈一谈他们的感受;当人们就某事发表意见时,会有一种能控制这个事物的感受,从而减轻他们的压力
    • 向他们提供尽可能多的信息;紧张往往是人们在缺乏信息的情况下下结论而造成的

YOUR RESPONSES

RESPONDING TO PEOPLE

- The customer is always right
- Seniors must be heeded
- Colleagues must be co-operated with

Responding to people at work can put you under pressure.
Try not to let your behaviour make it any worse.
Aggressive (fight) and submissive (flight)
behaviour will both increase the pressure.

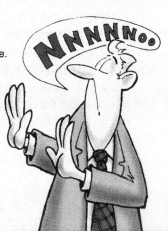

Use assertive behaviour instead. Learn to:

- Say 'no' to unreasonable requests and demands
- Reduce the pressure of conflict

对人的反应

- 顾客总是对的
- 对上级要服从
- 对同事要团结合作

在工作中和他人交往会产生压力,争取不要让自己的表现把事情搞得更糟。侵略性的行为(斗争)和服从性的行为(逃避)都会使你产生压力。

不妨采用肯定的态度。要学会:

- 对不合理的要求说"不"
- 减少由于矛盾造成的压力

RESPONDING TO PEOPLE

SAYING 'YES' WHEN YOU MEAN 'NO'

When...

- Everyone wants everything done yesterday
- Your day is just one interruption after another
- You feel that you're always 'fire-fighting'
- Your tasks remain untouched, while you deal with tasks for others

...you need to be proactive and say 'no'.

If you find it difficult to say 'no' try the **ADO** technique:

Acknowledge	show that you understand the request: 'So you want me to put the figures into a table that you can use in your presentation tomorrow?'
Decline	with a reason, but you don't have to explain yourself: 'I can do it, but not right now...'
Offer	an alternative: 'I can do it first thing tomorrow morning.'

你的反应
对人的反应
当你的意思是"不"时却说"是"

当处于下列情况时……
- 每个人都认为昨天就应该把所有事都做好了
- 你一天的工作总被人打断
- 感到自己总是在"救火"
- 在你的工作没有做的情况下,总是替别人处理任务

……你应该事先就打定主意,敢于说"不"

如果你觉得说"不"很难,可以试一试 **ADO**(确认—拒绝—建议)方法。

确认 表明你已明白了他的请求,"你是不是让我把这些数据填写在表格中,以便你明早口头报告用?"

拒绝 找一个理由,但你不一定要为自己解释:"我可以做,但现在不行……"

建议 给出选择:"明早第一件事就做它,怎么样?"

RESPONDING BY PLACING BLAME

CONTROL

Blame is a popular response to many of the pressures you face at work:

- You didn't get promoted, so you blame your boss
- You feel insecure in your job, so you blame the management
- You're late for a meeting, so you blame the previous one - it over-ran

Blame is an attempt to deflect the focus away from yourself. You use it when you feel threatened, insecure, alienated, out of control in some way. You use it when you're stressed. But it doesn't help.

你的反应
以责备的方式做出反应

    对工作中诸多压力的普遍反应是责备:
- 得不到提升时,责备自己的老板
- 工作中有危机感,责备管理不好
- 开会迟到了,责备上一个会议拖延太久

    责备是一种使注意的中心从自身转移的企图。当感到威胁、不安全,被别人疏远,或从某种程度上讲不能施加控制时,往往会发出责怨。紧张的时候也可能会责怪别人,但这样做不会有什么作用。

RESPONDING BY PLACING BLAME

In some situations, blame may bring you temporary relief from pressure in the short-term. It might, for example, 'buy you time' or turn the focus temporarily away from you. Perhaps you'll feel better pointing the finger at someone else and letting yourself off the hook. The relief is momentary. Having placed blame, you now have more pressures to contend with.

If you've used blame to:

- Cover a mistake, you worry that you may yet be found out
- Abdicate responsibility, it confirms your lack of control

If you want to avoid an increase in pressure, don't place blame.

你的反应
以责备的方式做出反应

　　在某些情况下,责备别人能使你暂时从压力中解脱,可以为你赢得一些时间或暂时引开别人对你的注意。也许当你把责任指向别人时,你会摆脱掉自己的责任,感觉会好一些。但这种解脱是暂时的。责备了他人之后,你会有更多的担心。
　　如果你责备:
　　• 是为了掩盖自己的错误,你会担心这早晚会被揭穿
　　• 是为了逃开责任,它证明了你缺乏控制事物的能力
　　所以你要是不想增加自己的压力,就不要责备。

RESPONDING TO CONFLICT

When you experience conflict at work do you:

- Avoid bringing attention to it in the hope that it will go away?
- Ask those involved in the conflict how they see the situation?
- Use status, authority or seniority to get what you want?
- Keep to the facts of the situation and avoid becoming emotional?
- Love it when you win and hate it when you lose?
- Select the best solution for everyone, or the solution you prefer?

The way you choose to deal with a conflict will determine how much stress it generates. Check your thoughts and responses. Do you increase the pressure when you deal with conflict or reduce it?

对冲突的反应

当你在工作中遇到冲突时,你的反应是:
- 希望冲突会自动消失,不去理睬它?
- 向卷入冲突的其他人咨询,看看他们对事情怎么看?
- 运用自己的地位、权力和资历得到你所要的东西?
- 根据实际情况办事,尽量避免冲动?
- 成功了则喜欢这件事,反之则充满了憎恶?
- 选择能让每个人都满足的解决方案,还是你喜欢的方案?

选择什么样的解决冲突的方法决定了这件事对你造成的紧张程度。核对一下你的想法和反应,你解决冲突的做法是增加还是减轻了你的压力?

RESPONDING TO CONFLICT
INCREASING THE PRESSURE

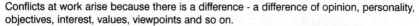

Conflicts at work arise because there is a difference - a difference of opinion, personality, objectives, interest, values, viewpoints and so on.

If you think of conflict in terms of a fight, a struggle, winners and losers, you may become defensive, aggressive, try to ignore it, or walk away from it.
These are all classic responses associated with stress.

Take a winners and losers approach to conflict and the losers will always:

- Have a desire for revenge
- Be inclined to bear a grudge

A winners and losers approach will simply encourage further conflict.
There will always be a 'sore point'.
It will fester. It will reappear.

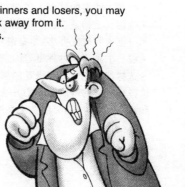

你的反应
对冲突的反应
导致压力增加

　　当人们在工作中意见有分歧,性格不同,目标不一致,兴趣、价值观和看问题的观点相左时就会产生冲突。

　　如果把冲突看成斗争,非胜则败,那么你就会充满防备、进攻的心理,对冲突不去理睬或避开。这些都是紧张时典型的反应。

　　对冲突持非胜则败观点的人,失败时往往会:

* 有报复的欲望
* 有怨恨的倾向

　　所以把冲突看成非胜则败的这种做法会导致更深的冲突。这个"痛点"会存在下去,会使人痛苦,不断出现。

RESPONDING TO CONFLICT
REDUCING THE PRESSURE

Try thinking of conflict as an opportunity to resolve differences, to reach a satisfactory solution for all, a chance to progress, to move forward, to improve working relationships and conditions. These perspectives are less likely to result in stress.

Take a win/win approach to conflict and you will reduce or eliminate pressure because:

- Everyone has a chance to be heard
- Working relationships and conditions are improved
- More trust and respect are generated
- Future conflicts become easier to confront

你的反应
对冲突的反应
使压力减轻

　　尽量把冲突看成是消除分歧、为大家找到满意的解决方案、促人进步、改善工作关系和工作条件的一次重要机会。这种想法往往不会导致紧张。

　　把冲突看成是一次双赢的机会，你就会减轻或消除压力，因为：

- 每个人的意见都可以得到倾听
- 工作关系和工作条件得以改善
- 更多的信任和尊重由此产生
- 将来的冲突解决起来也就容易多了

RESPONDING TO CONFLICT

THE LEAST STRESSFUL APPROACH

1. Acknowledge that conflict exists. Ignore it at an early stage and it will be much harder to resolve later.
2. Understand everyone's position. Listen to what is said. Restate each position to show that you've understood.
3. Identify key issues and concerns. Encourage honesty.
4. Search for possible solutions. Be creative. Be open minded. Don't evaluate or judge at this stage.
5. Select the best solution for everyone, not the solution you prefer.
6. Implement the solution and re-check that everyone is satisfied. If not, conflict will recur.

Always use language that is factual and neutral. Avoid emotion and blame.

This process is a series of stages. Each stage must be complete before moving on to the next one. Don't be in too much of a hurry. Haste might result in things being overlooked, people not being heard, people not having enough time to search deeply and to be honest.

你的反应

对冲突的反应

消除紧张的最佳途径

1. 承认冲突的存在。冲突初期得不到重视会为以后解决冲突带来难度。
2. 理解每个人的处境。仔细倾听别人的想法,重新表述一下每一个处境以确保你已听明白。
3. 找出最关键的问题和最大的忧虑。鼓励大家要真诚。
4. 寻找可能的解决方案。要有创造性。思想开放。在这一阶段先不要评判方法的好坏。
5. 选择对大家都有利的解决方案,而不是单凭你自己的喜好。
6. 实施解决方案,查看是否每个人对此方案都满意。要是有人不满意的话,新的冲突会出现。

总是使用切实的、中性的语言。避免情绪化和责备他人。

解决冲突的途径包括几个步骤。在没有完成上一个步骤之前不要开始下一步。不要急于求成。急躁会导致忽视某件事,有的人的心声没有得到倾听,解决问题的方法想得不周全,不完全真实可靠。

RESPONDING TO THE TRUE PRESSURE

When you realise that you're stressed and that you need to control your thoughts and responses to a pressure, make sure that you focus on the true pressure. Think carefully about it:

- Is your colleague really irritating you or are you actually concerned about your impending appraisal?
- Were you really so angry that the coffee machine wasn't working or was it just the last straw after a difficult meeting?
- Perhaps the pressure isn't even at work. Maybe it's at home and it just comes with you every day.
- Or, maybe the true pressure is you?

你的反应
对真正压力的反应

　　当你意识到自己紧张,需要控制自己对压力的想法和反应时,确保你关注的是真正的压力。要仔细考虑下列问题:
- 你的同事真的惹恼了你,还是你自己在为即将得到的评判而担心?
- 你是真的为咖啡机坏了而生气,还是它只不过是艰难会晤之后的导火索?
- 也许压力不是工作带来的,而是来自家庭,天天都伴随你左右?
- 或许压力的根源就是你本人呢?

PUTTING YOURSELF UNDER PRESSURE

You put yourself under pressure when you:

- Constantly strive for perfection
- Always put the needs of others first
- Lack self-esteem
- Blame others for your situation
- Dislike your job, but stay in it out of habit
- Try to please people all the time
- Say 'yes' every time you're asked to do something
- Carry your responsibilities all the time - never switching off

你的反应
给自己背上压力

当你有下列做法时,便给自己背上了压力:
- 总是力求完美
- 总是把别人的要求放在首位
- 缺乏自尊
- 为自己的状况去责备他人
- 不喜欢自己的工作,但出于习惯不愿改变现状
- 总想讨好别人
- 别人让你做事时总是说"好"
- 总是背负着责任——从不知放松

PUTTING YOURSELF UNDER PRESSURE

Try not to be so hard on yourself, and others. Reduce the pressure. You don't have to change your personality, just ease up a little from time to time.

Alternatively, you could say: 'That's just the way I am', 'I've always been like that', 'It's in my nature'. You could just carry on putting yourself under these pressures for the rest of your life.

Your pressure. Your response. Your choice. Your life.

你的反应
给你自己背上压力

不要为难自己和别人。减轻一下压力。你不必改变自己的性格,只要一点一点地放松自己就可以了。

或者你可能会说:"这就是我做事的方法","我一向就是这样","这就是我的本性"。那么你今后还会背负压力的重担。

你的压力。你的反应。你的选择。你的生活。

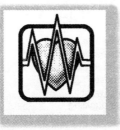

YOUR LIFESTYLE

你的生活方式

YOUR LIFESTYLE

LIVING WITH PRESSURE

Stress puts your body under pressure. It puts a
strain on your heart and your digestive system.
You become too busy or too tired to exercise
or to eat a balanced diet. You haven't got
time to relax and you really don't want
anyone else to know that you're buckling
under the pressure of work.

The way you lead your life can make you
more resilient to the pressures of work.
Or it can make the pressures worse.

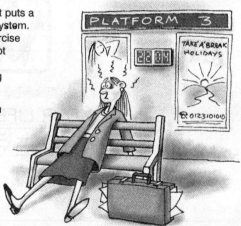

你的生活方式
带着压力生活

　　压力会使你的身体处于紧张状态,引起心脏和消化系统的紧张。你会因太忙太累而不能锻炼或平衡饮食。你没有时间放松,也不想让别人知道你在工作的压力下吃力地生活着。

　　你选择的生活方式或者使你在面对工作压力时更有弹性,或者加重你工作中的压力。

REGULAR EXERCISE

What happens when you see the words 'regular exercise'? Do you:

- Feel guilty because you know you should but...?
- Think you should turn to the next section because you're not the sporty kind?
- Think of exercise you used to enjoy before your life became so busy?
- Recall unhappy games lessons at school?
- Have visions of people who aren't at all like you?

You don't have to become a fitness fanatic, but you can build your defences against stress by improving your fitness.

你的生活方式
有规律的体育运动

当你看到"有规律的体育运动"这几个字时有什么反应？你是否有以下感受：

• 有负罪感，因为你知道应该锻炼，但……？

• 认为应该翻到下一章，因为你觉得自己不是一个运动型的人？

• 回想过去不像现在这么忙的时候你曾经喜欢的运动项目？

• 想到上学时烦人的体育课？

• 想象那些和你完全不同的人的样子？

你不必一定要做一个体育运动的狂热爱好者，但通过运动保持健康可以帮你克服紧张。

IMPROVING YOUR FITNESS

To improve your fitness, focus on the level, frequency and type of exercise.

Level of exercise
- Aim for a gradual steady improvement; if you don't walk anywhere, start walking.
- Become aware of your breathing; you are exercising at the right level when you have increased your breathing rate, but you're still able to speak to someone.

Frequency of exercise
- Too much exercise is as bad as too little.
- **Build up** to exercising on alternate days. Aim to exercise at the right level for periods of 20 to 30 minutes at a time. If you are starting from zero exercise, this will take several months to achieve. Don't expect too much of yourself too soon. A steady progression delivers results.

你的生活方式
增进健康

　　为了改变健康状况,要注意体育运动的强度、频率和类型。
运动的强度
- 要稳定地、逐步地提高强度;如果以前你从不步行,现在开始尝试步行出门。
- 注意呼吸。进行合适强度的体育运动时,呼吸加速但还能和别人讲话。

运动的频率
- 过多或过少的运动都不理想。
- 有规律地间隔**锻炼**可以增进健康。你的目标是每次选择合适的强度锻炼 20~30 分钟。如果以前你从未运动过,那么你要花上几个月的时间才能达到这个目标。不要期盼很快就有很大的成就。循序渐进会使你达到理想的效果。

IMPROVING YOUR FITNESS

Choose exercise that:

- You enjoy - exercise can be sociable or solitary, indoors or outdoors, at home or at a club.
- Will increase your rate of breathing.
- Is varied - sometimes swim, sometimes cycle, sometimes jog...
- Is not competitive to the point that it increases stress and defeats the object entirely!
- You can fit into your already busy life. Yes, it will take effort, but too much effort and you'll stop. Think about:
  - using the stairs at work
  - walking the block at lunch time
  - walking up the escalator
  - cycling to work
  - getting off the bus a little earlier and walking the last 15 minutes home in the evenings.

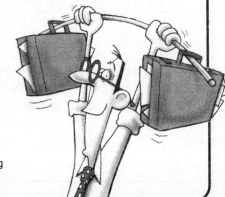

你的生活方式
增进健康

选择下列运动：

• 选择你喜欢的运动形式——运动可以是群体的，也可以是单独的；可以是户内的，也可以是户外的；可以在家运动，也可以在俱乐部运动

• 能使你呼吸加快的运动

• 不同形式的运动：游泳，骑单车，慢跑……

• 不会因竞争性过强而带来紧张以至于使你无法达到目标的运动

• 能在繁忙生活中进行的运动。运动确实需要努力，但若需要太多的努力，你就不会坚持运动了。你不妨考虑下列运动方式：

- 上班时爬楼梯

- 午饭时间在楼区散步

- 爬自动扶梯

- 骑车上班

- 下班乘车时提前下车，留下大约 15 分钟左右的时间步行回家

WHICH EXCUSE DO YOU USE?

Perhaps you:

- Haven't got time - just start to move more than usual; avoid the lift, take the stairs.

- Feel too tired - exercise will help you feel more energetic.

- Can't really be bothered - why not? Find out the real reason; this is a lame excuse!

- Feel you're too old - whatever your age you will benefit from improving your fitness. Just choose the right type, level and frequency to meet your needs.

- Haven't got anything to wear - don't confuse exercise with fashion. Many activities only require loose comfortable clothing. But do pay attention to your footwear. It should be comfortable, affordable and appropriate for the activity you've chosen.

选择什么样的运动？

也许你感到：

• 没有时间运动——那么你可以从现在做起，比平时多运动一些，不要乘电梯，自己爬楼梯

• 太累——那么运动会让你感到精力充沛

• 不愿很麻烦地去运动——为什么不愿去呢？分析一下原因，单说不愿意不是一个好理由

• 感到自己太老了——无论你年纪多大，只要选择合适的运动，进行强度适中、次数恰当的锻炼，都能增进健康，从中受益

• 没有合适的衣服穿——运动不是时装表演。很多运动只需要宽松舒适的衣服就够了，但一定要选择合适的鞋子。鞋子要穿起来舒服，价格适中，适合你所选择的运动

WHICH EXCUSE DO YOU USE?

Perhaps you:

- Have a bad back. Find out exactly what's wrong with your back; then seek advice on choosing an appropriate activity to strengthen the weakness you suffer from.
- Think it's boring. There are many ways to improve your fitness; choose one that you enjoy.
- Think you'll start when you've lost some weight - together with a balanced diet, exercise can help you to lose weight. Don't wait to lose weight before you start to exercise.

There is no real excuse for not improving your fitness. Start now. Don't be over-ambitious. Feel the benefits.

你的生活方式
选择什么样的运动?

也许你感到:

• 背部有毛病。那么先要查出背部有什么毛病,咨询该选择什么样的运动才能锻炼好自己的背部。

• 运动很枯燥。增进健康的运动方法有很多种,选一种你喜欢的。

• 等减肥后再运动。适当运动、合理饮食可以帮你减肥。不要等减肥后再去运动。

真正的运动都能帮你增进健康。现在就开始行动吧!野心不要太大,尽情感受运动的益处。

YOUR LIFESTYLE

LOOK AT IT THIS WAY

Think about how you feel when you're stressed.

Would it help if you could:

- Take your mind off things?
- Release tension?
- Feel better about yourself?
- Sleep more soundly?
- Clear your mind and relax?
- Feel more energetic?

Exercise gives you all these things. Try it.

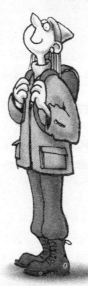

这样想一想

　　想一想紧张的时候你的感觉。
　　如果你能做到以下几点会不会感觉好一些？
- 不去想烦心的事？
- 释放焦虑？
- 觉得自己很棒？
- 睡得更好一些？
- 清空脑子，放松自己？
- 感到更加精力充沛？

　　运动能让你成功地做到以上几点。不妨试一试。

FOOD FOR THOUGHT

You would never consciously put the wrong fuel in your car.
Nor would you expect your car to run well on poor quality
fuel or to run without fuel. Why then do you expect your
body to function with the wrong type of fuel, poor
quality fuel or no fuel at all?

Because your digestive system slows down
and more acid is produced in the stomach
when you're under pressure, it's even
more important to be careful about
what you eat and when.

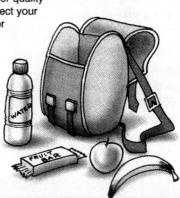

你的生活方式
饮食观念

　　你不会有意识地在自己的车里加不匹配的燃料,当然你也知道没有燃料或烧劣质燃料时车子是跑不快的。那么你为什么期望在使用不匹配的、劣质的燃料或根本就没有燃料时,身体还会继续工作呢?

　　一个人有压力的时候,消化系统运动变缓;胃里会产生过多胃酸,所以有压力时更要注意饮食搭配及进餐时间。

YOUR LIFESTYLE

CHECK THOSE HABITS

If when under pressure you...

- ...drink more coffee, try decaffeinated. Better still, drink water.

- ...smoke more, try asking colleagues to help you cut down.
  Buy something special with the money you save.
  Do something constructive with the time you save
  (moving away from your immediate area of work in
  order to smoke means that each cigarette takes at
  least 15 minutes out of your day).

- ...use alcohol to relax, try relaxing in other ways:
  take some exercise, do something
  with friends or family; spend time
  on a hobby.

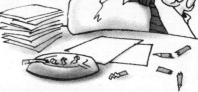

你的生活方式
检查自己的习惯

　　你若是在背负压力时……

　　• ……喝更多的咖啡,那么争取不要喝咖啡,喝水会好一些。

　　• ……吸更多的烟,那么要让同事帮你戒烟。用戒烟省下来的钱买些特别的东西。用节省下来的时间做些有意义的事。(离开工作出去吸烟意味着每根烟都要浪费你 15 分钟的时间。)

　　• ……用酒来放松,那么试试其他放松的方法:做运动,和朋友家人共同做事,做自己喜欢的事。

CHECK THOSE HABITS

If when under pressure you...

- ...just grab the nearest thing to eat, try to plan ahead. It will increase your chances of eating the right food and release you from the worry of where the next meal's coming from.

- ...skip lunch because you're too busy, try taking a short break to eat something. Paradoxically, taking a break will improve your concentration. You will work better.

- ...eat more comfort foods, try eating figs, dates or other dried fruit when you need something sweet. Whilst chocolate and other comfort foods may give you a temporary lift, a short time later, you will feel worse than before.

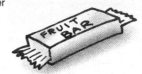

- ...end up having to eat late in the evening, choose something light and easy to digest.

检查自己的习惯

　　你若是在背负压力时……

　　• ……有什么就吃什么,那么就要学着事先安排饮食。这样可以使你合理饮食并解除对下顿饭吃什么的担心。

　　• ……因为太忙而不吃午饭,那么应该休息一下,吃点饭。休息会提高你的注意力,虽然这看上去矛盾,实际上千真万确。你能更好地工作。

　　• ……吃更多的安慰食品,那么当你想吃甜食时,不妨试试吃些无花果、海枣或其他干果。虽然巧克力和其他的安慰食品会使你暂时振奋,但不久之后你会感觉更糟。

　　• ……搞到很晚才吃饭,那么要吃些清淡的、易消化的食物。

ARE YOU TENSE OR RELAXED?

When you're stressed your muscles will be tensed
in readiness for action. Unless released, this
tension becomes a source of discomfort.
Your:

- Head thumps and you can't think straight

- Eyes are sore and tired

- Body aches

The way to release this tension
is through relaxation.

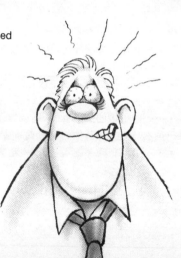

你是紧张还是放松?

当一个人紧张的时候,肌肉也会紧张,以便做出反应。除非能及时释放这种紧张,否则这种紧张会令人感到非常不舒服。

紧张时你会:
- 头脑昏沉,不能有条理地思考
- 眼睛疲劳疼痛
- 身体疼痛

只有通过放松才能释放这些紧张。

ARE YOU TENSE OR RELAXED?

Be aware of the tensions in your muscles when you're at work. Release them.

- Are your legs crossed tightly? Place your feet flat on the floor.
- Is your brow furrowed? 'Smooth' it.
- Where is your tongue? Release it to the floor of your mouth.
- Return your shoulders to their natural position.

Doing something that really makes you laugh also works well. When did you last laugh?

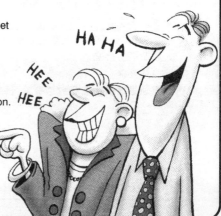

你的生活方式

你是紧张还是放松?

工作时要意识到你的肌肉是否紧张。紧张的话,一定要放松。

• 看看你的腿是不是在紧张地交叉着?如果是,把你的双腿平放到地板上。

• 你的眉毛是不是在紧锁着?如果是,把它们舒展开。

• 你的舌头在什么位置?让它放松,平放在嘴底部。

• 把肩头舒展到自然的位置。

做一些真正使你发笑的事也会有很好的效果。你最近一次大笑是在什么时候?

RELAXATION FOR THE EYES

Working at a computer screen or VDU console, reading for long periods, working in very bright or very dim lighting can strain your eyes. Straining your eyes can lead to sore eyes, irritability, headaches and fatigue. Regularly relaxing your eyes with the following technique will help to reduce the strain.

Read through the following steps several times to familiarise yourself with them. Then try the whole exercise.

1   Sit with your head squarely on your shoulders and widen your eyes as much as you can.
2   Keep your head still and raise your eyes to look towards the ceiling. Hold this position for a slow count of 5.
3   Now roll your eyes slowly round to your right. Focus on something and hold it for a slow count of 5.
4   Keeping your head still, roll your eyes down, focus and hold for a slow count of 5.
5   Now roll your eyes to the left, focus and hold for a slow count of 5.
6   Roll your eyes upwards again and repeat in the other direction.
7   Finally close your eyes, let your head and shoulders relax and rest for a few moments.

你的生活方式
眼部放松

在电脑屏幕前或 VDU 演奏台前工作,长时间读书,在太强或太弱的灯光下看书都会使眼睛疲劳。眼睛疲劳会导致眼睛酸痛,出现过敏反应、头痛和疲劳。以下放松眼睛的技巧会帮你解除眼部的疲劳。

把下列步骤读上几遍,记住它们,然后再做整个练习。

1. 正坐。眼睛尽可能睁大。
2. 头部保持不动,眼睛往上看天花板。保持这种姿势慢慢数到 5。
3. 现在眼睛慢慢往右转,集中看某个地方,保持这种姿势慢慢数到 5。
4. 头部保持不动,眼睛慢慢往下转,集中看某个地方,保持这种姿势慢慢数到 5。
5. 现在眼睛慢慢往左转,集中看某个地方,保持这种姿势慢慢数到 5。
6. 再把眼睛往上转,然后重复刚才其他方向的几个动作。
7. 最后闭上眼睛,头和肩部放松,休息几分钟。

RELAXING COMPLETELY

Take some time out at home and try to relax completely. Read through the steps below several times to familiarise yourself with them. Now put them into practice:

- Take the phone off the hook; switch your mobile phone off; tell your family that you don't want to be disturbed

- Lie down on a bed or the floor with your feet apart and palms facing upwards

- If you do need to support your head, use a slim pillow - the flatter you are the better

- Close your eyes and, starting from your feet, work your way around your body, focusing on each part, making sure it is relaxed before moving on to the next part

- When you first do this, your mind will wander; don't worry because with practice your mind will wander less and relaxation will be achieved more easily

Once you start to experience the benefits of relaxation try other ways such as massage, yoga, visualisation, meditation, the Alexander Technique. Find a class to go to or use some of the many books, audio tapes and video tapes available to help yourself.

你的生活方式
全身放松

　　在家里花些时间,试一试全身放松。把下列步骤读上几遍,记住它们。现在你就可以试一试了:

- 把电话机摘下来,把手机关掉,告诉家人不要打扰你。
- 躺在床上或地上,双腿分开,掌心朝上。
- 如果你需要支撑头部,也可以枕一个小枕头——总之你躺得越平越好。
- 闭上眼睛,从脚开始放松,注意力依次集中到身体的各个部位,在转到下一个部位前,确保这个部位已经放松。
- 刚开始做的时候,你肯定会走神,不要担心;因为随着不断练习,你的思想会越来越集中,越来越容易放松。

　　当你感到放松的好处后,还可以尝试推拿、瑜珈、想象法、药物疗法或亚历山大法等其他方法。参加培训班或买一些书、磁带、录像带等帮自己放松。

THE VALUE OF SUPPORT

When you're under pressure the support of others is invaluable. Talking your situation through can help to:

- Clarify your thoughts
- 'Get it off your chest'
- Put things in perspective
- Sort out real from imagined issues
- Give you a different perspective
- Reduce the sense of isolation that pressure can generate

Others may be a source of guidance, direction or information; they may motivate, inspire or renew your enthusiasm. Maybe you know this, but you still don't seek their help because:

- You don't want to appear unable to cope
- You're concerned that asking for help is seen as a weakness
- Your request for support might be refused

The solution is to know how to ask, when to ask and who to ask.

134

他人帮助的价值

   当你面对压力时,别人的帮助是无价之宝。把你的困境讲出来会帮你:
- 理清自己的思路
- 把烦恼倾诉出来
- 恰当地处理问题
- 把真实存在的问题和想象中的问题分开
- 给你提供分析问题的新思路
- 减少压力带来的孤独感

   别人能给你提供指导方向和信息,他们可以激励、鼓舞、重新激发你的热情,你也清楚这些,但你还是不愿意去寻求帮助,这是因为:
- 你不想表现出对付不了这件事的样子
- 你担心寻求帮助会被别人看成软弱
- 你的请求有可能被拒绝

   克服这些担心的方法是学会如何请求帮助,在何时请求帮助,以及找谁来帮助你。

ASKING FOR HELP

1. How to ask

- State your concern. Be factual, be specific: 'I'm concerned about the increase in my workload, since we reorganised the department'. Avoid dramatisation: 'I've got work coming at me from all sides. I just don't know where to turn next. I'm at my wit's end'.

- Say what you want. Do you want guidance, an opinion, inspiration, a listening ear? Remember, it's support you're seeking; you should not expect others to solve your problems.

- Ask when it would be convenient. Showing respect for someone else's time reduces the chances of an outright refusal of your request.

2. When to ask

Sooner rather than later. If you leave it too long, both asking for and giving support becomes more difficult.

请求帮助

1. 如何请求帮助

• 说清你的担心。要属实,具体,例如:"自从我们这个部门重组以来,我就担心工作负荷的增长。"不要夸张,例如:"我不得不对付来自各方面的工作。下一步该做什么我都不知道。我已经黔驴技穷了。"

• 说出你想要什么。你需要指导、意见、鼓励还是倾听? 切记,你是在寻求帮助,不要指望别人帮你解决全部问题。

• 询问什么时候方便去请教。尊重他人的时间安排,可以减少被马上拒绝的可能。

2. 什么时候去请教

越早越好,如果时间拖延太长,对于请求帮助和提供帮助的人来说都会很困难。

ASKING FOR HELP

3. Who to ask

Think about what you want and then ask the most appropriate person. Consider asking associates, colleagues, seniors, people outside the organisation.

It's unreasonable to expect one person to provide all your support so build yourself a network of supporters. The most effective networks are those that provide a balance of give and take. If you support others, they are more ready to return the favour when you're in need.

Plan time to build and maintain rapport with your contacts. Being in touch with them only when you need help makes a weak network.

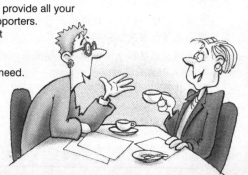

请求帮助

3. 请谁帮助你

决定你想要什么之后，找一个合适的人去请教。不妨向伙伴、同事、资深的人、公司外的人去请教。期盼一个人能给你提供全部帮助是不大现实的，所以你要自己建立一个支持你的关系网。最有效的互助关系网是那种既有得到又有付出的组织。如果你帮助了别人，在你需要帮助时，他们也会主动伸出援助之手。

花些时间和你认识的人建立并保持良好的关系。当你需要别人时才保持联络会使联络网变得很脆弱。

FINDING TIME TO ADAPT

Adapting your lifestyle so that you're more resilient to the pressures at work will take time. Time is something that you might not have when you're under pressure, so think about focusing on something that:

- **Creates time:** How much time do you spend in front of the TV flicking from channel to channel, hoping that there will be something to entertain you? Try watching just one programme less in a week. You'll free up an hour. What will you do with that hour?

- **Doesn't take time:** If time is a real pressure for you at work, stop wearing a watch at weekends. Try it. Eat when you're hungry. Go to bed when you're tired. Ignore the time. Take the pressure of time right out of your life. It makes a difference.

找时间适应

　　调整你的生活方式,以便能更有弹性地适应工作中的压力,这要花费一些时间。当你处于压力中时,可能会感到没有时间。所以考虑一下集中精力做某些事,它能够:

　　• **创造时间**:有多少时候你是坐在电视机前从一个频道换到另一个频道,希望会有些好的节目看? 一周试着少看一个节目,你就会多出一个小时。这一个小时你将会做什么?

　　• **不考虑时间**:如果时间在你的工作中确实是个压力,周末时你就不要戴手表。试一下。饿的时候再去吃饭。累的时候才去睡觉。不去注意时间。把时间的压力从你的生活中赶出去。这样会有所不同。

GETTING STARTED

Changing your lifestyle is a challenge. Use these tips to get you started:

- Be realistic; start with something small and build on it
- See the solutions, not the obstacles
- Don't make too many changes at once or changes that are too big
- Make a commitment to yourself; write reminders and actions in your diary
- Re-live your achievements; make notes of your progress at the end of each week and re-read them
- Accept that you're human; even if your resolve occasionally weakens, stick with it
- Create a reward system for yourself
- Start now; get results - tomorrow may be too late

开始行动

改变生活方式是一个挑战。运用下列建议会让你开始行动：

- 现实些，从小的方面开始并逐渐发展
- 要看到解决的方法，而不是障碍
- 不要一下子做太多太大的变化
- 给自己做一个承诺；在日记里写下提醒和行动
- 再次体验你的成就；每周末把你的进步记下来，再读一读
- 接受你是凡人的事实，即使偶尔你的决心受挫，也要坚持下去
- 给自己制定一个奖励机制
- 从现在开始；收获结果——明天就可能太晚了

GETTING RESULTS

收 获 结 果

THE THREE ESSENTIALS

Managing stress at work is easier said than done.

To get results you need to:

- Recognise stress
- Know how to apply first aid
  (what to do in the short-term)
- Aim to prevent rather than cure
  (a long-term view)

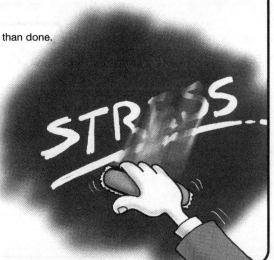

三个基本点

要控制工作中的紧张,说起来容易,做起来难。

要收获结果,你需要:

- 认知紧张
- 知道如何运用首选求助方法(短期内要做什么)
- 旨在预防而不是治疗(从长远观点来看)

CHOOSE TO RECOGNISE IT

Stress is a downward spiral. If you choose to ignore it:
- You become less able to cope
- The problems get worse
- The pressures increase

As a consequence:
- You suffer more stress
- The situation becomes more complex
- Seeking help becomes more difficult
- Getting back to 'norm' requires excessive amounts of time and effort

Do you have plenty of time and effort to spare?
What shape are you in? Can you afford to be stressed?

选择认知它

紧张呈恶性发展。如果你选择忽视它：
- 你会变得更没有能力对付它
- 问题会恶化
- 压力会增加

结果是：
- 你更加遭受紧张之苦
- 情况变得更复杂
- 更难以寻求帮助
- 恢复到"正常"状况需要更多的时间和精力

你有大量的时间和精力吗？

你处于什么状态？你能受得了紧张吗？

WHAT SIGNS WILL YOU LOOK FOR?

The quicker you recognise stress, the easier it is to manage. Nip it in the bud.

What signs will you look for?

Think about physical, mental, emotional and behavioural signs.

What might you see, hear or feel?

What's the earliest warning signal your body gives you?

Is it always the same one?

你要寻找什么样的迹象?

你越早认知紧张,控制起来就越容易。把它扼杀在萌芽状态。

你要寻找什么样的迹象?

想一想身体上、精神上、情绪上和行为上的迹象。

你会看到、听到或感到什么?

你身体最早发出的警告信号是什么?

总是同样的信号吗?

MENTAL FIRST AID

THEORY

Think about it.

Your body is giving you signals that you're stressed.

Why?

Because you've triggered the fight or flight response.

Why?

Because you perceived a situation as a threat or a challenge.

Thinking about the situation in a different way can check the downward spiral of stress.

精神上的首选求助

理论

考虑一下。

你的身体发出信号表明你处于紧张状态。

为什么?

因为你激发了迎击或逃离反应。

为什么?

因为你把某种情况看做是威胁或挑战。

用一种不同的方式来考虑这种情况会制止紧张的恶性发展。

MENTAL FIRST AID

PRACTICE

Try turning your mind to something else:

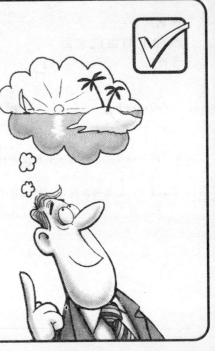

- Daydream for a few moments
- Use self-talk ('I won't get angry, it's not worth it; I'll just state my case again, calmly')
- Think how much worse the situation could be
- Keep an open mind (you're reacting badly to what you've just overheard; resolve to keep an open mind until you've established the facts)
- Check your attitude - is it positive?

You have the mental power to check the fight or flight response. Use it.

精神上的首选求助

练习

试着想点别的事：

• 做一会儿白日梦

• 自我交谈（"我不生气，它不值得我生气；我会平静地再次申明我的情况"）

• 想一想情况有可能会坏到什么地步

• 保持头脑开放（为刚才无意中听到的事你就反应得如此强烈；在事实确凿之前，要下定决心保持心胸开阔）

• 检查一下你的态度——它是积极的吗？

你拥有能制止迎击或逃离反应的精神力量。运用它。

PHYSICAL FIRST AID

THEORY

When you perceive a threat or challenge, your body automatically goes into a state of alert.

Ignoring these signs means that you are in a permanent state of preparation.

The body's natural instinct is to go on trying to adapt under increasing pressure. Unless you stop it, your body will eventually break down.

Making a physical change can help your body revert to its norm.

收获结果
身体上的首选求助
理论

当你察觉到威胁或挑战时,你的身体会自动进入警觉状态。

忽视这些迹象意味着你将长期处于备战状态。

身体的自然反应会尽力适应增加的压力。除非你阻止这一趋势,否则身体会最终崩溃。

在身体方面改变一下会帮你的身体恢复到常态。

PHYSICAL FIRST AID

PRACTICE

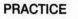

How is your body responding?

- If your breathing has become shallow, breathe slowly and deeply
- If your body is tensed, release the gripped muscles
- If you're slumped or slouched, sit or stand tall

Try it. It makes you feel different, doesn't it?

Can you physically walk away from the situation? Can you quite literally take a break?

Smile. Do it now. Feeling stupid doing it? Make your smile wider. Laugh at yourself. Feel different? Yes, the pressure's still there, but with that small action you've given the signal for your body to return to norm which is what first aid is all about. The sooner you apply it, the quicker you'll see results.

身体上的首选求助

练习

你的身体是怎么反应的？
- 如果你的呼吸变得短促,那么缓慢地深呼吸
- 如果你的身体紧张,那么把绷紧的肌肉放松
- 如果你的身体弯垂、懒散,那么就要站直或坐直

试一试。它会使你感觉不同,是不是？

你能否离开当前的状况？你能去彻底休息一下吗？

笑一笑。现在就这样做。感觉这样做很傻吗？笑得再厉害些。自己对着自己笑。感觉到不一样了吗？是的,压力还在,但就是这么一个很小的动作,就给了你的身体一个信号,让身体恢复到正常状态,这就是首选的求助方法。你越早运用它,就能越快收到效果。

SCEPTICAL ABOUT FIRST AID?

Why?

Stress is caused by what happens in your mind and your body. It starts with a thought that turns into a physical response.

The way to stop it is to counter that thought and check that response.

You have a choice. You can choose to:

- Think and respond in a way that will **increase** your stress

  OR

- Think and respond in a way that will **reduce** your stress

收获结果

怀疑首选求助方法?

为什么?

紧张是由精神和身体发生的变化造成的。它源于思想,继而转变为身体上的反应。

阻止它的办法是遏制这种思想,制止身体的反应。

你有一种选择。你可以选择:

• 以**增加**你的紧张的方式思考和反应

或者

• 以**减轻**你的紧张的方式思考和反应

BUT ISN'T FIRST AID DIFFICULT?

Thinking and responding in a way that will reduce stress can be difficult when you're under pressure. Positive thoughts and positive actions are often the last things on your mind.

But unless you think positive and act positive, you'll simply spiral downwards.

You are the only one who can break that spiral. No one else can do it for you. You may not have full control over the pressures around you, but you do have full control over your thoughts and responses. You can choose to think and respond negatively. You can choose to think and respond positively.

收获结果
但是使用首选求助方法不也很困难吗?

当你背负压力时,以一种减轻紧张的方式思考和反应确实很困难。积极的思考和行动往往是你最不愿想的事。

但除非你积极地思考和行动,否则你将彻底卷入恶性发展的漩涡。

你是唯一能阻止情况恶性发展的人。没人能替你去做。你也许不能完全控制困扰你的压力,但你能完全控制你的思想和反应。你可以选择消极地思考和反应。你也可以选择积极地思考和反应。

THINKING POSITIVELY

Thinking positively will make you more positive. It becomes a self-fulfilling prophecy.

When you need to apply first aid try to:

- Push negative thoughts away as soon as they come into your mind
- Avoid people who are negative and destructive
- Focus on something positive to occupy your mind
- Think about known, proven facts only
- Be objective
- Use a mental mantra ('I will...'; 'I am...'; etc)
- Remind yourself that everything is relative
- Avoid reading things into a situation
- Stay rational
- Focus on what you've achieved (even when it feels like nothing, there will always be something)

DON'T make excuses. Take action. Get results. Use first aid techniques to regain control.

收获结果
积极地思考

积极地思考可以使你更积极。它会成为自我实现的预言。

当你运用首选求助的方法时,应努力做到:

- 脑子里一有消极的想法,就马上把它们赶走
- 避免接触消极和有负面影响的人
- 集中精神想积极的东西
- 只考虑已知的经证明的事实
- 要客观
- 运用精神咒语("我将……""我是……"等等)
- 提醒自己一切都是相对的
- 不要在某一环境中做无中生有的推断
- 保持理智
- 注重你取得的成绩(即使你好像没有取得过什么,但你总有过某项成绩)

不要找理由。采取行动。收获结果。运用首选求助的方法恢复控制。

PREVENTION RATHER THAN CURE

THEORY

While first aid has a vital role to play in managing your stress at work, the fact that you need to apply it means that you are already experiencing stress. You've already triggered the fight or flight response.

Each time you trigger the response, you put your body under a greater strain. In your bid to handle the pressures you're under, you turn a blind eye to your body's signals. You fail to see that your performance has become impaired. You push your body too far. It gives you aches and pains, ulcers and heart attacks. It breaks down.

Where stress is concerned, prevention is preferable to cure.

收获结果
预防而不是治疗
理论

　　尽管首选求助的方法对于控制工作中的紧张有重要作用,但你需要运用它这一事实说明你已经处于紧张状态了。你已经激起了迎击或逃离反应。

　　每当你激起这种反应时,你的身体就处于一种紧张状态。在你试图对付自己的压力时,却对身体发出的信号不加理会。你没有看到你的表现已经退步了。你把自己的身体搞得太累。它会使你觉得疼痛,产生胃酸和犯心脏病,这样身体会崩溃。

　　对紧张,预防比治疗要好。

PREVENTION RATHER THAN CURE

PRACTICE

To prevent stress you need to stop triggering the fight or flight response.

How many times in a normal working day do you unwittingly initiate it?

- An accident on the route to work means you arrive late
- Your colleague is sick, so now you have to fill in
- The phone rings incessantly
- Everyone wants the job done yesterday
- The boss wants to see you now
- Your 'to do' list remains untouched

The aim of stress management is to reduce the number of times you trigger the fight or flight response. It requires certain skills.

收获结果
预防而不是治疗
练习

　　要想预防紧张,你需要制止迎击或逃离反应。

　　一个正常工作日中你有多少次不明智地激起迎击或逃离反应呢?

- 路上的事故意味着你上班迟到
- 你的同事病了,所以现在你不得不临时补缺
- 电话铃响个不停
- 每个人都希望工作在昨天就已经做好了
- 上司现在要见你
- 你的任务单上的工作还未动

控制压力的目的在于减少你激起迎击或逃离反应的次数,这需要一定的技能。

GETTING RESULTS

PREVENTION SKILLS

Learning not to trigger the fight or flight response requires a combination of skills. These skills may be:

- **Mental**   Adjusting your perspective; using positive self-talk
- **Physical**   Relaxing; improving your fitness
- **Organisational**   Balancing the workload; making more of your time
- **Behavioural**   Being assertive; managing conflict

Stress is an individual's response to pressure. What skills do you need to prevent stress? Use the pages in the 'Your Thoughts' and 'Your Responses' sections to give you ideas.

收获结果
预防技能

　　学会制止迎击或逃离反应需要综合技能。这些技能是:
- **精神上**　　调整你的观点;积极地自我交谈
- **身体上**　　放松;增进健康
- **组织上**　　平衡工作量,更充分地利用时间
- **行为上**　　果断;控制冲突

　　紧张是个人对压力的反应。你需要什么技能来防止紧张?阅读"你的想法"和"你的反应"章节,以得到一些想法。

SCEPTICAL ABOUT PREVENTION?

Why?

- **Because you've read the book, seen the video, attended the training course?**
  Maybe you know about prevention skills in theory. Maybe from time to time you even put them into practice. But do you do it consistently? Prevention skills are about thoughts and responses that you use naturally in the course of your work. They're habits.

- **Because you haven't got time?**
  There's no doubt that learning to prevent stress takes time. But do you have the time to recover from stress-related illnesses? Can you afford to be off work?

收获结果
不相信预防作用？

为什么？

• 因为你已读过书,看过录像,参加过培训课程？

也许理论上你对预防技能有所了解,也许时不时会在实际中运用它。但你坚持这样做了吗？

预防技能是你在工作过程中自然而然产生的想法和反应。它们是习惯。

• 因为你没有时间？

毫无疑问,学习预防紧张需要花时间。但你有时间去治疗与紧张有关的疾病吗？你承受得起不上班工作的代价吗？

SCEPTICAL ABOUT PREVENTION?

Why?

- **Because it sounds like hard work?**
  Breaking old habits and developing new ones does involve effort. But what's the alternative? As the saying goes: *'If you always do what you've always done, you'll always get what you've always got'*.

Being sceptical about prevention skills will only add to your pressure. If you have concerns, try looking at them in a different light.

收获结果
不相信预防作用？

　　为什么？
　　· 因为它听起来好像是件艰难的工作？
　　打破旧的习惯，形成新的习惯确实需要努力。但是有其他的选择吗？俗话说："如果你总是做已经做过的事，那么你就总是收获你已经得到的东西"。
　　对预防技能的怀疑只会增加你的压力。如果你还存有担心，试着用不同的观点来看它们。

CONCERNED ABOUT TIME?

If you're concerned about the time that adopting prevention skills will take, remember that:

- Prevention skills are about stopping as well as starting things. Find something that you need to stop doing. Free up some time. Use it to develop your stress prevention skills.

- While you're fretting about it, you're actually wasting time. Stop fretting. Think and do something positive.

- When your prevention skills have become habits, you will actually have more time.

收获结果

担心时间?

　　如果你担心采用预防技能会花去你的时间,记住:

　　• 预防技能意味着停止做某些事,以及开始做某些事。找出一些你需要停止做的事,空出这些时间,用它来发展你预防紧张的技能。

　　• 当你为它而烦躁时,实际上你在浪费时间。不要烦躁了,考虑一下,做些积极的事。

　　• 一旦预防技能成为习惯,你就会拥有更多的时间。

MAKE THE RIGHT CHANGES

Developing prevention skills means making changes. Before initiating a change, make sure it's worth it. Some changes turn out to be additional sources of pressure.

Avoid:

- The flavour of the month change:
  Last month it was 'The Grapefruit Diet', this month it's 'Bananas and Pears.'
  You will fail to make progress.

- The hot air change:
  You talk constantly about getting a new job, but don't even start the process.
  You will lose face.

- The half-baked change:
  You stop smoking, but start over-eating.
  You will lose your self-esteem.

收获结果
做正确的改变

发展预防技能意味着进行改变。在你开始实施某项改变之前,确信它值得你去做。有些改变最后会成为新的压力来源。

避免:

• 频繁的改变

上个月你用"葡萄减肥法",这个月是"香蕉和梨"。

这样你不会有进步。

• 说大话的改变

你不断地说要去找份新工作,却总不行动。

你会丢面子的。

• 草率的改变

你停止了吸烟,却开始暴食。

你会失去自尊。

MAKE THE RIGHT CHANGES

Avoid:

- The cart before the horse change:
  You enter yourself for the local marathon, and then take up jogging.
  You will over-stretch yourself.

- The damp squib change:
  You manage two days with no coffee, but now you're back on the usual drip feed.
  You will become irritable - and that's a sure sign of stress.

All these changes increase the pressure you're under. Only make changes that reduce your pressure.

收获结果
做正确的改变

避免:

• 次序颠倒的改变

你报名参加地方的马拉松比赛,然后才开始慢跑。

这样会使你过分紧张。

• 无成效的改变

你坚持两天没喝咖啡,但现在你又得靠静脉注射度日。

你变得易怒——这肯定是紧张的迹象。

所有这些改变都会增加你背负的压力。应只做那些能减轻你压力的改变。

PLANNING WORTHWHILE CHANGES

Ask yourself four questions to ensure that you don't even begin to make a change until you've established that it will be worthwhile.

Consider:

1. What you do now?
2. What you want to do?
3. How you're going to do it?

Then ask yourself:

4. Is it worthwhile?

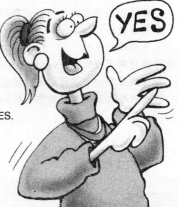

Adjust your plan until the answer to question 4 is YES.
Only then will you get results.

收获结果
为值得的改变做计划

问自己下列四个问题来保证在确定改变值得与否之前,不轻易做出改变。
考虑一下:
1. 你现在正在做什么?
2. 你想做什么?
3. 你打算怎么做?
然后问自己:
4. 它值得做吗?
调整你的计划直到你对问题 4 的回答是"是的"。只有到那时,你才能收获结果。

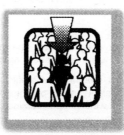

STRESS IN YOUR ORGANISATION
组织中的紧张

YOUR ROLE & RESPONSIBILITIES

Stress is an individual's reaction to pressure. The individuals in an organisation are therefore responsible for stress at work. Everyone is responsible.

When people at work are stressed, morale is low, inefficiencies abound, mistakes are made, absenteeism rises, profits fall. When an organisation suffers from stress, it starts on the same downward spiral that we experience as individuals.

As an individual within an organisation you should take the responsibility to manage your own stress and:

- Ensure that you're not a source of pressure
- Help others who are under pressure
- Encourage a low stress culture

你的职位和你的责任

　　紧张是个人对压力的反应。因此在组织中的个人要对工作中的紧张负责。每个人都负有责任。

　　当人们在工作中处于紧张状态时,士气低落,效率低下,出现错误,缺勤增加,利润下降。

　　当一个组织遭受紧张之苦时,它也会像人一样,呈恶性发展趋势。

　　作为组织中的一员,你应该负起控制自己紧张的责任,并且:

- 确保你不是压力的来源
- 帮助那些处于压力之中的人
- 鼓励一种低紧张度的文化

ARE YOU INCREASING THE PRESSURE?

We're all human. We all have faults. But have you ever considered that when you think you are...

- Working well as a team member
- Being a good leader
- Helping others

...you may actually be increasing the pressure?

你在使压力增加？

我们都是人，我们都会犯错。但是你是否想过当你认为你……

- 作为小组一员工作做得很出色时
- 是一个好领导时
- 在帮助别人时

……实际上你可能在使压力增加？

STRESS IN YOUR ORGANISATION

BEING A SOURCE OF PRESSURE

Pressure on others is increased by:

- Being inconsistent - blowing hot and cold
- Letting people down - not doing what you said you would do
- Imposing your own values - if you work through lunch breaks and at weekends, you expect others to do this too
- Not planning - always being in a last minute rush and needing something done 'yesterday'
- Being aggressive or submissive rather than assertive
- Being unnecessarily 'loud' in a shared work area
- Taking a negative perspective
- Being possessive about equipment, work or information that others would benefit from
- Being overly competitive and always needing to 'win'
- Ignoring the feelings or needs of others
- Interrupting

 Do you do any of these things? Are you a source of pressure for others?

成为压力的来源

他人的压力会因为下列原因而增加：

- 前后不一致——出尔反尔
- 使别人失望——没有履行诺言
- 把自己的价值观强加于人——如果你在午餐时间和周末仍继续工作,你希望别人也这样做
- 没有计划——总是在最后一刻还在匆匆忙忙并需要某些事在"昨天"就做好了
- 好斗或惟命是从;不果断
- 在一个共同工作场所不必要地"大声说话"
- 持有消极的观点
- 不愿意与别人分享能使他们受益的设备、工作和信息
- 竞争心过强并总想要"赢"
- 不顾别人的感情和需求
- 打断别人

你有上述行为吗? 你是别人压力的来源吗?

STRESS IN YOUR ORGANISATION

BEING A SOURCE OF PRESSURE

Ironically, many of the things listed opposite increase the pressure on you too.
Stop doing them. It will help to reduce your pressure and the pressure within your
organisation.

What else do you do that might increase pressure?

Find out by talking to the people you work with. Ask them what you can stop doing to
reduce pressure at work.

- **B**e prepared to take it on the chin
- **A**ct on it right away
- **C**heck that the change has reduced the pressure
- **OFF**er to do something else

If you're a source of pressure at work, **BACk-OFF**.

成为压力的来源

　　具有讽刺意义的是,上页列出的很多项同样也会增加你的压力。不要做这些事了。这样将有助于减轻你和你组织内部的压力。

　　你还做了什么其他可能增加压力的事?

　　和同事谈谈,把引发压力的事情找出来。问问他们如果要减轻工作中的压力,你需要停止做哪些事。

- 做好承受痛苦的准备
- 马上行动
- 核实你的改变是否已经减轻了压力
- 主动做些其他事

如果你是工作中压力的根源,那么就**消除**它。

PRESSURE IN THE TEAM

As a member of a team you are part of a group that has been formed solely for the convenience of the organisation. The only thing you may have in common with other team members is a set of goals. How do you behave in your team?

Do you:

- Work as an individual rather than a team member?
- Withhold information from others in the team?
- Break into sub-groups rather than work together?
- Indulge in win/lose conflicts within the team?
- Pursue your own agenda rather than the goals of the team?
- Fail to pull your weight?

If you are doing any of these things you are creating pressure for yourself and others. Stop. If others are behaving in this way, confront them and resolve it.

团队中的压力

　　作为团队中的一员,你是小组的一分子,小组仅仅是为了组织的方便建立起来的,你和团队中其他成员唯一共同的东西是一系列的目标。在团队中你表现如何?

　　你是否:

- 作为个体而不是团队中的一员在工作?
- 隐瞒信息,不告诉团队中的其他成员?
- 又分成几个小组而不是整个团队共同工作?
- 在团队中沉溺于输/赢的纷争?
- 追求个人安排而不是团队的目标?
- 没有干好本职工作?

　　如果你有上述表现,你就在给自己和别人增加压力。不要这样做了。如果别人有上述行为,正视他们并解决这个问题。

WHEN YOU'RE IN CHARGE

When you are in charge of others at work, reduce the pressure on yourself by:

- Taking 'time off' from your responsibilities; leave work and leave it behind

- Delegating - in the short-term it may seem time *consuming but in the long-term it's liberating*

- Creating time to think and plan, to step away, rather than do

- Accepting that you will not always be liked by everyone

- Having a degree of humility

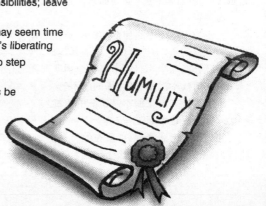

While the nature of your job may not enable you to do all of these things all of the time, try doing at least one of them every day.

组织中的紧张

当你是主管时

在工作中,当你管理别人时,通过下列方法减轻自己的压力:

- 从你的职责中抽出一点时间;离开工作,忘掉它
- 委托——从短期来看,它可能会消耗时间,但从长期来看,它可以解放你的时间
- 抽出时间思考、计划,先不工作,暂时走开
- 接受你不可能被每个人都喜欢这一现实
- 保持一定程度的谦恭

尽管你的工作性质可能使你无法做到这一切,试着每天至少做其中的一件。

BEING RESPONSIBLE FOR OTHERS

When you're responsible for others at work reduce pressure on them by:

- **Motivating with a carrot rather than a stick**

  Both the stick and the carrot will increase pressure. But the stick is more likely to be seen as a threat. As such it's more likely to trigger stress. Try not to use it.

- **Making any criticism constructive**

  Be specific. State the problem in terms of the behaviour not the person. Agree a course of action.

- **Avoiding knee jerk, dictatorial styles of management**

  Participative, open, empowering styles are generally less stressful.

对别人负责

  当你在工作中负责管理他人时,可以通过下列方法减轻他们的压力:

• 用胡萝卜而不是大棒激励别人

  胡萝卜和大棒都会增加压力。但是大棒往往更被视为一种威胁。因此更有可能引发紧张。尽量不要使用它。

• 使批评具有建设性

  要具体。阐述问题时对事不对人。同意某种特定情况下的做法。

• 避免机械的、命令式的管理方法

  参与、开放、授权等领导方式带来的紧张通常会少一些。

BEING RESPONSIBLE FOR OTHERS

When you're responsible for others at work reduce pressure on them by:

- **Encouraging a culture that reduces pressure**

  Make it acceptable to take lunch breaks and holidays. Don't make people feel guilty if they're the first to leave work. Talk openly about stress.

- **Getting to know them**

  Learn to recognise their individual signs of stress and what might cause them stress. Their signs, concerns and values may be very different from your own.

- **Making it easy for them to ask you for help**

  Avoid the macho attitude of 'if you can't stand the heat get out of the kitchen'. The longer a situation is left before it is aired, the more complex it may become. It may, therefore, be more difficult to resolve.

组织中的紧张
对别人负责

当你在工作中管理他人时,可以通过下列方法减轻他们的压力:

• **鼓励能减轻压力的文化氛围**

允许有午饭休息时间和假期。如果有人第一个下班,不要让他感到有负罪感。公开坦然地谈论紧张。

• **逐步了解他们**

学会辨认他们每个人紧张的迹象和可能会引起他们紧张的那些事。他们的迹象、担心和价值观可能和你的有很大不同。

• **使他们的求助方便容易**

避免大男子主义的态度,"如果你不能忍受厨房中的热气,就不要呆在厨房里"。问题越晚公开提出,它就会变得越复杂,也就可能越难解决。

WHEN YOU'RE ASKED FOR HELP

When someone asks you for help they're already under pressure. Try not to increase it further.

DON'T:

- ✗ Dismiss their concern - 'You're probably worrying over nothing'
- ✗ Give your opinion unless you're asked for it
- ✗ Question their actions - 'Why on earth did you do that?'
- ✗ Be judgmental - 'I certainly don't think you should have...'
- ✗ Hijack the conversation so they can't get a word in
- ✗ Relay your own life history - 'That sounds like when I was at...'
- ✗ Give sympathy - give empathy instead

Doing any of these things will probably:

- ● Leave someone feeling worse than before
- ● Increase the pressure they're under
- ● Discourage them from seeking help in the future

当别人向你求助时

当有人向你求助时,他们已经处于压力之中。尽力不要让这种压力增加。

不要:

✕漠视他的担心——"你可能在为不存在的事担心"

✕给出自己的意见,除非别人要你发表意见

✕质问他们的行为——"你究竟为什么要那么做?"

✕做出判断——"我当然认为你不应该……"

✕强占谈话以至于他们无法插话

✕转述自己的历史——"这听起来像是当我在……"

✕给予同情——而要给予共鸣

做以上任何事情都可能:

• 让某人感觉比以前更糟

• 增加他们承受的压力

• 使他们灰心,今后不愿寻求帮助

HOW TO HELP OTHERS

When you're giving help to others:

DO:

1. Let them speak

✔ Give them time; don't hurry them; be prepared for silence
✔ Encourage them with open questions - How? When? Where? Who? What?
✔ Extend their comments - 'Tell me more about...'
✔ Use supportive statements - 'I see...' 'Okay' 'That's interesting...'

2. Listen to them

✔ Use body language to show that you're listening -
eye contact, nodding, raising of eyebrows
✔ Show that you are following by saying 'mm', 'right' 'uhha'
✔ Reflect back what's been said - 'So you feel that...'
✔ Check that you understand - 'So your main concern is...'

组织中的紧张

如何帮助别人

当你帮助别人时：

要：

1. 让他们讲话

√ 给他们时间；不要催促他们；对他们的沉默要有准备

√ 用开放式的问题鼓励他们——怎样？什么时候？哪里？谁？什么？

√ 鼓励他们多评论——"多讲一些关于……"

√ 使用支持性的语言——"我明白了……""好""那很有意思……"

2. 听他们说话

√ 使用身体语表示你在倾听——目光接触，点头，挑眉毛

√ 通过说"嗯""对""啊"来表示你在听他说话

√ 对刚才说的话给予反馈——"所以你觉得……"

√ 核实一下你已经理解了——"所以你主要担心的是……"

HOW TO HELP OTHERS

When you're giving help to others, **DO:**

3. Help them to help themselves
   By doing this they will learn how to handle similar situations and cope better in the future. Help them to:
✔ Establish what the real problem is
✔ Explore different perspectives
✔ Seek solutions by asking 'what if' questions

4. Follow-up
✔ Find out how they're getting on. Check that they're making progress.

Important
- DON'T try to solve their problems for them or 'rescue' them
- DO consider getting them to read this book
- If you feel that someone needs more than first level assistance with stress management, encourage them to seek the guidance of a fully trained stress counsellor or therapist

如何帮助别人

当你帮助别人时,**要**:

3. 帮他们学会自助

这样做可以使他们学会如何应付类似的情形,在将来做得更好。帮他们:

√ 确认真正的问题是什么

√ 探寻看问题的不同角度

√ 通过问"要是……"这样的问题来寻求解决方案

4. 后续工作

√ 看看现在他们做得怎么样。核实他们正在进步。

重要的是:

• 不要试图为他们解决问题或"营救"他们

• 一定要考虑一下请他们读读本书

• 如果你感到控制紧张的初步帮助对某些人还不够,要鼓励他们从受过全面培训的顾问或精神治疗专家那里寻求帮助

ENCOURAGING A LOW-STRESS CULTURE

Everyone in an organisation contributes towards its culture. To create a low-stress culture it is important to:

- Take responsibility; don't be part of a blame culture
- Talk about stress; make it acceptable rather than taboo
- Avoid linking your self-esteem to your earning power or holding promotion as an emblem of success
- Learn as much as you can about stress and put it into practice
- Communicate, keep people informed; if you don't know, ask
- Co-operate; work together
- Give and accept support
- Learn to accept change

Stress is catching, make sure you're not the one that's spreading it.

鼓励低紧张度的文化

每个人对组织文化都会有一定的作用。为了营造一个低紧张度的文化,重要的是:
- 承担责任,不要成为责备文化的一部分
- 谈论紧张,让人们接受它而不是忌讳它
- 不要把你的自尊和收入能力联系起来,或把提升看成是成功的象征
- 尽可能学习有关紧张的知识并将其付诸实践
- 交流,让人们得到信息;不了解信息就问
- 合作,共同工作
- 给予并接受帮助
- 学会接受变化

紧张是会传染的,确保你不是传播紧张的人。

YOUR FUTURE

Everyone experiences pressure, and pressure at work often results in stress. But it doesn't have to. While you may not have the ability to control all the pressures you face, you do have the ability to control your responses to them. Use this ability. Your relationship with stress depends on it.

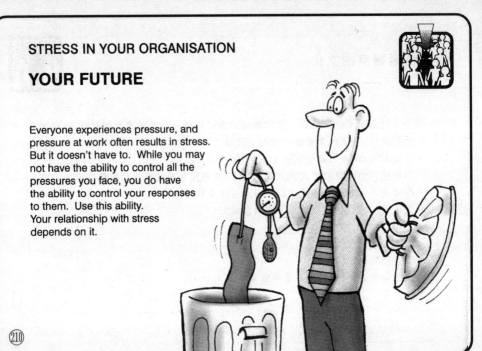

你的未来

　　每个人都会经受压力,工作中的压力往往会导致紧张,但并不是一定如此。虽然你可能没有能力控制你所面对的所有压力,但你的确有能力控制你对压力的反应。要运用这种能力,你与紧张的关系是由此决定的。

About the Author

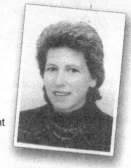

Mary Richards BEd, MCIM, is a business consultant and trainer with a background in education, international marketing and general management. She has her own training and consultancy business, and her clients include both private and public sector organisations.

Combining her education and training skills with her management experience, Mary also writes business skills publications and resource materials for trainers. She is the author of 'The Telephone Skills Pocketbook' in this same Series.

To reach Mary Richards, please contact the publisher in the first instance.

Published by:
Management Pocketbooks Ltd.
14 East Street, Alresford,
Hants SO24 9EE, U.K.
Tel: +44 (0)1962 735573
Fax: +44 (0)1962 733637
E-mail: pocketbks@aol.com
Web: www.pocketbook.co.uk

All rights reserved

This edition published 1998. Reprinted 1999

© Mary Richards 1998

ISBN 1 870471 62 8

Printed in U.K.

作者简介

　　玛丽·理查德　教育学士、特许管理学院成员、商业顾问和培训员。主修教育、国际市场和一般管理。拥有自己的培训和咨询公司。她的客户既有个人,也有政府资助的企业。

　　玛丽拥有丰富的教育知识,也拥有管理经验中积累的培训技巧,所以她也编写了商业技能手册和培训素材类丛书。

　　要联系玛丽,请先与出版社联系。

出版社:

管理袖珍丛书有限公司

公司地址:英国 汉普郡

　　　　　阿尔瑞斯彼德区

　　　　　东大街 14 号

　　　　　SO24 9EE

电话:+44 (0) 1962 735573

传真:+44 (0) 1962 733637

电子邮箱:pocketbks@aol.com

网址:www.pocketbook.co.uk

ISBN　1 870471 62 8

于英国印刷

读者意见反馈卡

谢谢您购买本书,请您填妥下表,以便我们今后为您提供更好的图书。

书名:《英汉对照管理袖珍手册;缓解紧张》

请填写(或附名片):

姓名: 邮编:

E-Mail: 电话:

年龄: 职业:

地址:

1. 您认为本书采用英汉对照的方式对您的学习有帮助吗?

   有 没有

2. 您希望本书采用何种方式?

   全部中文 全部英文 英汉对照

3. 认为本书翻译质量如何?

   很好 尚可 较差

4. 您从何处购得此书?

书店　　邮购　　商场　　其他:＿＿＿＿＿＿＿

5. 您是如何得知本书的?(请在画线处写上报纸或杂志的名称)

书店　　朋友　　报纸:＿＿＿＿＿＿＿＿　　杂志:＿＿＿＿＿＿＿

其他:＿＿＿＿＿＿＿

6. 您喜欢本书的封面吗?

喜欢　　　　　　　　不喜欢

7. 您认为本书的价格:

偏高　　　　　　　　中等　　　　　　　　偏低

您的目标价位是:＿＿＿＿＿

8. 您认为本书的翻译有重大错误吗? 如果有,请填写或用其他方式与我们联系:

＿＿＿＿＿＿＿＿＿＿＿＿＿＿＿＿＿＿＿＿＿＿＿＿＿＿＿＿＿＿＿＿＿

＿＿＿＿＿＿＿＿＿＿＿＿＿＿＿＿＿＿＿＿＿＿＿＿＿＿＿＿＿＿＿＿＿

如有任何疑问和要求,请与我们联系:

上海交通大学出版社　　　　　　　　　电话:021-61675269

地址:上海市番禺路 951 号　　　　　　邮编:200030

电子邮箱:wangliatcn@gmail.com(邮件主题请写丛书名或书名)

联系人:汪俪

英汉对照管理袖珍手册(第1辑)

1	思维技巧	☐	14	面谈高手	☐
2	提高效率	☐	15	做个培训者	☐
3	时间管理	☐	16	新员工培训	☐
4	团队合作	☐	17	绩效管理	☐
5	激励	☐	18	商务计划	☐
6	决策	☐	19	管理变革	☐
7	会议事务	☐	20	做个管理者	☐
8	个人成功	☐	21	项目管理	☐
9	人员管理	☐	22	评估管理	☐
10	缓解紧张	☐	23	影响力	☐
11	资产负债表	☐	24	问题行为	☐
12	现金流管理	☐	25	商务演讲	☐
13	预算管理	☐			

英汉对照管理袖珍手册(第 2 辑)

英汉对照管理袖珍手册(第 3 辑)

本丛书可在当当、卓越、京东等网店购买。

1. 如需邮购,请将汇款寄至:

　上海市番禺路 951 号,上海交通大学出版社读者服务部　收

　邮编: 200030　　　　　　电话: 021-61675298

　请在汇款留言中写明所购图书品种以及数量。国内邮寄免收邮费。

2. 也可在书名后的方框内填上购买册数,传真至读者服务部。

　传真: 021-64071208

已推出盒套装(50 种),定价:550 元